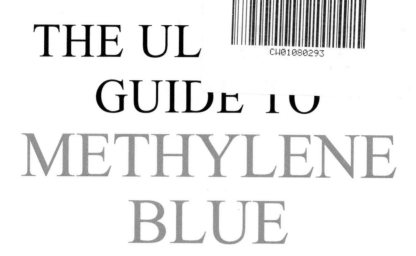

THE UL GUIDE TO METHYLENE BLUE

Remarkable Hope for Depression, COVID, AIDS & other Viruses, Alzheimer's, Autism, Cancer, Heart Disease, Cognitive Enhancement, Pain & The Great Transition to Metabolic Medicine

MARK SLOAN

A proud presentation of:

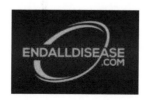

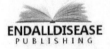

Published by Endalldisease Publishing
ISBN (Paperback): 978-1-998284-00-9

DISCLAIMER

DISCLAIMER

This book does not claim to treat, cure, heal, assess or reverse a disease, addiction, ailment, defect, injury, or psychological condition. The information contained within this book should not be used to diagnose, treat or cure any medical condition, illness, disease, metabolic disorder, or health problem of any kind. The information presented herein is for educational purposes only and is not intended as medical advice. If you have a medical problem, or suspect you have one, contact your physician or health care provider. Also, be sure to consult your physician or health care provider before beginning any nutritional or exercise program. Neither the author nor the publisher assumes any liability for any injury, illness or adverse effects caused by the use or misuse of the information contained herein. Under no circumstances will any legal responsibility or blame be held against the publisher or author for any reparation, damages, or monetary loss due to the information in this book, either directly or indirectly. The reader is solely responsible for the use of the programs, advice and other information contained in this book.

Table of Contents

Introduction

My book *Bath Bombs and Balneotherapy* hit shelves last year, and the response so far has been tremendous. I want to say thank you personally to everyone on the EndAllDisease *Advanced Readers Club* who picked up a free pre-release copy of the book and left an honest review on Amazon. As long as you keep the reviews coming in, I'll be happy to offer you pre-release copies of all future books.

Writing and publishing books has been the most challenging thing I've ever done; I've heard it aptly compared to "overcoming a disease." It's definitely a form of self-sacrifice but hearing how my work is helping people makes the struggle worthwhile. In the interest of keeping the good news flowing, I decided to jump right back into the fire and write another book. Unsure what to write about next, I asked my readers what they would like to learn about.

The four options for book topics were Acne, Prostate Cancer, Breast Cancer, and Methylene Blue. Here are the results of the survey…

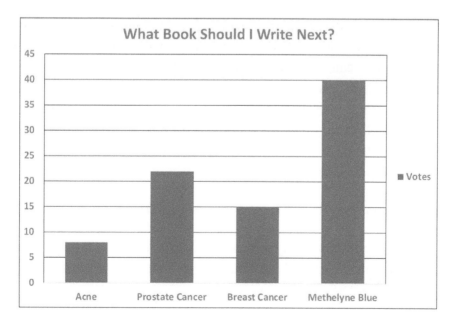

As you can see, the overwhelming majority of people selected methylene blue. In fact, it won by a landslide. The interesting thing is that most people who chose methylene blue didn't know what it was, other than it was a type of metabolic therapy, in some ways similar to red light therapy.

It's clear that people are yearning for practical solutions to disease and ready to move on from the failed genetic-based treatment paradigm and onto medicines that target the metabolism. Is methylene blue one of these medicines? Should people reach for methylene blue when they fall ill with a common cold? And can methylene blue tackle some of the more serious diseases, like Alzheimer's, Diabetes, or Cancer? These are just some of the many questions that I'll answer in the pages to come.

This book constitutes the third in a series documenting safe and effective metabolic therapies. Red Light Therapy and Balneotherapy were the first two, and I'll complete the trilogy with this book on Methylene Blue.

After establishing the foundations of high-quality metabolic medicine, I'll use that information to begin tackling each individual disease, dispelling the myths about their origins, warning people about any potential dangers associated with mainstream drug and surgical interventions, and then establishing evidence-based treatment protocols that can be used to heal the mitochondrial dysfunction underlying the disease.

It is a pleasure to present to you this work about the medicinal blue dye methylene blue. It's taken almost a year to write and has truly been a labor of love. I hope you enjoy reading it and thank you for supporting my work.

The Dye that Needs No Introduction, but Here's One Anyways

Want to revitalize the washed-out fabric of your favorite blue shirt? Any blue dye will do. But there's one dye in particular –

methylene blue – that could put you on the fast track to better health by adding a few drops to a glass of water or your favorite juice.

Of course, we will discuss the specific details in later chapters. First, I'd like to give you a basic understanding of the history of methylene blue and an introduction to the many things it could potentially do for you.

What is Methylene Blue?

Methylene blue is an inexpensive blue dye developed by scientists in the 19th century for the textile industry. In addition to being a brilliant blue dye for fabric, surprisingly, it was soon discovered to be useful in the scientific laboratory and in medicine. As a stain, it could help scientists see bacteria, parasites, yeasts, and other microorganisms when looking under a microscope. By adding the blue dye to microorganisms on an imaging plate, the internal structures and tiny organelles are illuminated and more easily seen by scientists. Remarkably, methylene blue is such a reliable stain that scientists still use it today in laboratories worldwide. But a stain for microscopy is only the tip of the iceberg as far as what methylene blue can do for science and the world.

Keeping the Fish Healthy

Fish hobbyists and fish farmers routinely use methylene blue as a treatment for keeping their fish and aquatic ecosystems healthy. Methylene blue is considered a safe aquarium disinfectant for marine life and is a robust anti-fungal and anti-parasitic agent. It is also used to treat fish eggs to ensure they are not lost to fungal overgrowth.

Anybody who has ever had a fish tank knows how delicate aquarium ecosystems are, which is a testament to the safety of methylene blue. Methylene blue can be used to treat some specific fish disorders, including nitrite poisoning, ammonia poisoning, swim bladder disorder, and general fish stress.

Dogs, Cats, Horses, Cows, and Pigs

Although not specifically approved for veterinary use, veterinarians commonly use methylene blue on numerous types of animals for treating methemoglobinemia[1] and other chemical poisonings. Later, I will summarize the existing research on methylene blue for various animals so you can see which conditions it might be effective for and a dose that appears to be safe and effective.

An Antidote for Chemical Poisonings

Most people today don't know that if you overdose on a pharmaceutical or street drug, swallow some toothpaste containing the insidious poison fluoride, or eat a poison mushroom, methylene blue is the first line of treatment doctors and nurses will administer in an emergency. In fact, methylene blue is an effective antidote for virtually all chemical poisonings. Also used for drug overdoses and chemical poisonings in hospitals are activated charcoal and sodium bicarbonate, also known as baking soda, which I've written about extensively in my book *Cancer: The Metabolic Disease Unravelled.*

Malaria Cured in 48 Hours

Methylene blue was the first antimalarial drug ever used in medicine and successfully treated all types of Malaria in the late 19th and early 20th centuries. Methylene blue works by inhibiting the Malaria-causing parasite *Plasmodium falciparum*, including drug-resistant types. Since then, methylene blue has been replaced with other antimalarial drugs, and for some time, had been forgotten. But a recent revival in methylene blue research for Malaria has shown that it could be the *most effective* antimalarial drug ever developed.

Viruses Don't Stand a Chance

According to the research, many of the viruses that the public is taught to fear are quickly inactivated by methylene blue, including Herpes, West Nile, Hepatitis C, Ebola, Zika, HIV, and COVID-19. And perhaps the most promising part is the startling increase in anti-microbial potency of methylene blue when combined with light therapy. It turns out, the combination of methylene blue and specific wavelengths of red and near-infrared light poses an even more significant threat to the survival of all types of pathogens and harmful microorganisms. We'll look in-depth at methylene blue's potential to treat viral infections in an upcoming chapter.

A Brain-Boosting Powerhouse

We all have days when our brain function feels slow, unfocused, and foggy. Can methylene blue help improve brain function and cognition, including parameters such as memory retrieval, attention, and emotional regulation? There's a growing body of evidence that suggests it can. Whether you want to be more productive, more emotionally stable in your relationships, or improve your ability to remember names, dates, or other facts and figures, methylene blue could potentially be a game-changer for you.

Goodbye, Depression

Since the announcement of the COVID-19 pandemic in March 2020, decreased human interaction seems to have become a more-or-less permanent feature of our lives. These changes essentially mimic the behavior of people who are depressed, which explains why depression is at an all-time high. And given that existing anti-depressant drugs from pharmaceutical companies (SSRIs) often come with debilitating and sometimes life-threatening side effects, never has the world been more in need of safe and effective remedies for alleviating the root cause of depression.

Recent research has shown that a single dose of methylene blue can completely eliminate symptoms of depression in some individuals. From my experience testing dozens of different drugs and nutrients over the past 15 years for their effects on my own depression, nothing has had a more positive impact on my life than methylene blue. If somebody is avoiding the social interactions necessary to live without depression, ultimately, their behaviors will need to change for permanent resolution. However, methylene blue might be a great option for you until you forge those meaningful relationships and connections.

Forget Dementia

When I was a child, my grandfather suffered from Parkinson's disease. Near the end of his life, he couldn't walk, talk, or survive without constant care 24 hours a day by my grandmother. I remember watching him being rolled into our living room in his wheelchair to spend time with the family, knowing that he had no idea who any of us were. I still feel sad when I think about it. And the reality is there are probably millions of people right now who are suffering the same fate after slipping into mental oblivion like my grandfather. Their loved ones pay the price by having to spend all their time caring for them. What would it mean for society if we could alleviate this suffering and need for constant care?

Recent research has shown that methylene blue can powerfully target the hallmarks of brain aging that can be found in pathologies like Alzheimer's and Parkinson's. These diseases share the common feature of mitochondrial dysfunction and repairing dysfunctional cellular metabolism is methylene blue's specialty. Imagine the improvement in the quality of life – for individuals, families, and society – when people with dementia are suddenly able to remember their loved ones' faces and retain their autonomy again. Soon I'll take you on a guided tour of the research on methylene blue for dementia.

Cancer Cells Are Targeted First

One of the most remarkable things about methylene blue is that it selectively targets the cells most in need of healing first before others. Any cells which stray from the highly efficient form of energy metabolism called oxidative phosphorylation, including Cancer cells, are selectively targeted and restored by methylene blue. This means that the sicker a person is, the more beneficial and profound methylene blue therapy will likely be.

Methylene blue therapy for Cancer has been studied far more than you might think, and we will go over the fascinating body of research in an upcoming chapter. Directly alongside red light therapy and balneotherapy, methylene blue therapy represents one of the most promising metabolic interventions for resolving the dysfunctional metabolism seen in Cancer.

Highly-Efficient Energy Storage

One surprising yet fascinating development in methylene blue research is its exceptional ability to store energy and then release it on command. These characteristics are ideal for someone seeking to develop an efficient battery for storing electricity, which is exactly what researchers have invented.

Remarkably, the methylene blue battery operates at a near-perfect efficiency. And when compared to batteries you'll find at your local store, methylene blue batteries are non-pollutant, more efficient, and much less expensive to manufacture. The superior efficiency and non-toxicity of organic methylene blue batteries could revolutionize how the world stores and delivers energy.

Dysfunctional Metabolism No More

One of the most remarkable scientific discoveries in recent decades is that over 90% of diseases that exist today are metabolic in nature. In other words, no disease pathology can be looked at independently from metabolism. This means that for virtually all diseases, including Cancer, the genetic component has been vastly overestimated. From a practical sense, what this means is that if somebody in your family has or had a certain disease, you are in no way destined to develop it – and many times, you're not even at increased risk at all. It is your hands on the steering wheel.

Since virtually all diseases are metabolic in nature, understanding how the body's metabolism works and maintaining its efficient function is the key to health and longevity. When cells are unable to use oxygen, methylene blue can act like the missing enzyme, which quickly restores oxidative metabolism. This basic action can explain the long list of healing benefits methylene blue can offer – all with practically no negative side effects. It's not difficult to see why the World Health Organization has added methylene blue to its list of Essential Medicines.[2]

One Last Thing...

My overall goal in writing this book was to create the most complete resource ever written on the subject of methylene blue. I want to help as many people as possible get the quality information they need to become knowledgeable and confident enough to make their own health decisions.

This book was designed to help you decide whether you want to add methylene blue to your medicine cabinet by giving you a thorough understanding of the existing scientific and clinical evidence showing what it can do. I hope this book will serve as a timeless and invaluable resource in the decades, even centuries, to come.

Once you're finished reading, please take a few minutes to write a quick and honest review on Amazon. I read every review personally, and I use the feedback to make improvements to the book in future editions.

If you haven't already, be sure to subscribe to my newsletter at Endalldisease.com, where you'll receive all the latest books and articles that I publish, as well as three free eBooks just for signing up.

Strap yourself in for this adventure into the fascinating world of dye therapy. Let's go!

PART I:
Nitric Oxide &
The Origins of
Disease

Nitric Oxide:
Miracle Molecule or Aging Accelerant?

"A theory that is wrong is considered
preferable
to admitting our ignorance."
– Elliot Vallenstein, Ph.D.

Our story on methylene blue begins in a place you might not expect—looking at a molecule often hailed for its 'miraculous benefits.' Unbeknownst to most of its advocates, it is actually a toxic component of air pollution, called nitric oxide (NO).

While writing this, I am reminded of the famous 1984 film *The Karate Kid*, in which the very first Karate lesson Mr. Miyagi taught to his student Daniel was how to wash and wax a car. In future lessons, Daniel was taught how to sand the floor, paint fences, and catch flies with chopsticks. Not surprisingly, Daniel was confused about why he was being taught skills that seemed entirely unrelated to Karate. But in time, Daniel realized that everything had a purpose. Mr. Miyagi's unique brand of martial arts taught Daniel important lessons like muscle memory, patience, focus, and precision that he would later use to become a master at his craft.

Similarly, there's no way that you can fully comprehend or appreciate methylene blue without first understanding the role of nitric oxide in health and disease and how it relates to the body's metabolism. This is why I've dedicated Part 1 of this book to nitric oxide and the origins of disease. Once you grasp the physiological role of nitric oxide in the body, the reason why the methylene blue dye is a shining star among medicines will become clear. So, sit back, relax, grab a cup of coffee and enjoy the ride.

How the Drug Viagra Flipped Nitric Oxide Research on its Head

In the 1980s and prior, the compound nitric oxide was well-understood by scientists to be a toxic free radical found in city smog. Then suddenly, according to Dr. Raymond Peat, around the year 1990, publishing activity in scientific journals began occurring in droves, claiming that nitric oxide was not only safe, but highly beneficial for an endless list of applications, including erectile function, heart function, and as a stroke preventative. In 1992, nitric oxide was proclaimed "Molecule of The Year."[1] The high volume of research and acclaim for nitric oxide around this time lead to the FDA approval and launch of the drug Viagra (sildenafil) for the treatment of erectile dysfunction, in 1996. "Viagra came out, and suddenly the medical publications came out finding it was the most glorious protective substance," said Peat. The pharmaceutical companies had succeeded in convincing scientists and the public at large that nitric oxide was no longer a toxic free radical but a miraculous healing substance that could improve human health in a myriad of ways, solely to market and reap enormous profits from their latest blockbuster drug.

But what does Viagra have to do with nitric oxide, you might ask?

Prescribed to millions of men for erectile dysfunction, Viagra acts by elevating nitric oxide levels in the body. Put simply, Viagra is a nitric oxide agonist. Such is the link between nitric oxide and the erection drug Viagra. But how could boosting nitric oxide be beneficial for the sexual health of men when it is known to decrease the fertility hormone testosterone?[2] And if nitric oxide is so helpful for cardiovascular health, then why is the nitric oxide *inhibitor* L-NAME "beneficial in the treatment of patients with refractory cardiogenic shock"?[3] Lastly, why does lowering nitric oxide provide a "striking survival benefit" in lung Cancer[4], and pancreatic Cancer patients[5]?

Type "nitric oxide" into a search engine, and you'll be inundated with studies and information from scientists, doctors, and the multitude of companies selling nitric oxide supplements and prodrugs, touting NO as a miracle material with a virtually endless list of benefits. You might also notice that around 95% of the information that emerges on the first few pages of any search engine regarding nitric oxide colors it in a positive light that would make the reader think it is one of the most health-promoting substances available. But buried deep within the digital trash heap known as the internet, there exists no shortage of evidence to the contrary, which in my opinion, is far more compelling and scientific.

In this chapter, I'm going to make the case that nitric oxide is not the health panacea that drug company researchers and marketers of nitric oxide-promoting supplements would have you believe. My position is that nitric oxide is part of the body's stress response fundamental to the aging process and virtually all chronic degenerative diseases, including Diabetes, Cancer, Heart Disease, Stroke, and Dementia. If this chapter casts even a modicum of skepticism onto your preconceived notions about nitric oxide, then it has succeeded. Softening our beliefs and admitting we could be wrong is the essential first step to learning anything new and moving in the direction of truth.

If the information I'm about to present conflicts with your beliefs about nitric oxide, I ask that you keep an open mind about it. If you find yourself feeling angry at any point, let me remind you that we cannot make any scientific progress when we don't allow ourselves to explore new ideas. Try the information on like you would try on a new jacket. This seems like a good place to drop a quote from one of the great philosophers from years past.

"It's the mark of an educated mind to be able
to entertain a thought without accepting it."
– Aristotole

With that in mind, and in the spirit of curiosity, I present to you the case against nitric oxide.

Nitric Oxide: A Toxic Free Radical

Nitric oxide is a signaling molecule that's produced naturally by the human body, and it is also present in the Earth's environment in the form of industrial pollution. Chemically, nitric oxide is a colorless gas and a free radical. What's a "free radical"? I'm glad you asked.

A free radical is any molecule that has an unpaired electron, which means that it's highly reactive with other chemicals and cellular structures inside the body. Virtually all known toxic environmental chemicals are free radicals as well, including heavy metals like lead, aluminum or arsenic, plastic compounds like bisphenol a, ionizing and non-ionizing radiation emitted by baby monitors, internet routers, cell phones, and X-rays, as well as the litany of different deleterious chemicals found in drugstore soaps, shampoos, and deodorants, like sodium lauryl sulfate.

"Free radicals are basically nasty little chemicals that go around stealing electrons off other molecules in your body, and that causes damage in the body," describes Dr. Emma Beckett, molecular nutritionist at the University of Newcastle in Australia. A balance between free radicals and antioxidants in the body is necessary for proper physiological function. Excessive concentrations of free radicals can overwhelm the body's ability to neutralize them and contribute to diseases like Cancer, heart disease, cognitive decline, vision loss, and virtually all other disease pathologies.

In 1956, after noticing that the concentration of free radical oxidants in the body gradually increases with age, scientist Denham Harman proposed *The Free Radical Theory of Aging*. Harman's theory suggested that free radicals cause damage from cumulative oxidative stress, resulting in aging and death. Currently, the evidence backing up this theory is so widespread that at this point, most scientists see the association as self-evident. In a 1998 review of the research on the free radical theory of aging, nitric oxide was labeled, "a damaging oxidant." It was said that the nitric oxide synthase (iNOS) – the primary enzyme that stimulates nitric oxide production – must be seen as "a potential source of damaging oxidants." Also mentioned by the scientists was the fact that "NO reacts with $O_{-2}\cdot$ to form peroxynitrite (ONOO−), itself a powerful oxidant."[6]

The opposite of oxidants like nitric oxide are antioxidants. "Antioxidants are the only things that can give up an electron to that reaction without becoming free radicals themselves. So they're halting that negative chain reaction,"[7] stated Dr. Beckett. Said differently, antioxidants selflessly donate an electron to oxidants, which prevents them from stealing an electron from healthy cells or tissues. The result is that the body is chemically stabilized. Vitamin C and vitamin E are two examples of antioxidants that can protect us against environmental chemicals, but you already knew that. One less commonly-known example of an antioxidant is urea, found in urine.[8] This is why, for thousands of years, as described by the Roman poet Ovid, women have been splashing mule urine on their faces to promote more youthful skin. (Think that's gross? Take a look at the ingredients list on the bottle of your face cream. If it's a quality product, it probably contains urea).

To sum things up in one sentence: free radicals cause damage, and antioxidants protect against damage. As with most things, any excess can cause harm, so once again, *balance* is the key.

Let's return to our subject of nitric oxide now. Given the fact that most people are exposed to an excess of free radicals daily in the form of environmental chemicals in food, water, air, plastics, and drugstore personal care products – does it sound like a good idea to further increase free radicals in the body by taking nitric oxide-promoting drugs or supplements like Viagra or L-arginine?

Nitric Oxide for Bodybuilding

For decades, the bodybuilding world has been promoting nitric oxide for its ability to dilate or relax constricted blood vessels, claiming "an increase in nutrient and oxygen delivery means you'll be able to exercise for longer, no matter what your sport is," wrote Casey Walker on his blog *Myprotein*. An article on bodybuilding.com offers "6 Vein-Popping Reasons To Use Nitric Oxide Supplements", including:

1. Increased Recovery Rates
2. Reduced Fatigue Levels During Higher Rep Protocols
3. Enhanced Endurance Performance
4. Increased Availability of Energy
5. Increased Glucose Use
6. Increased Muscle Pump

All these benefits sound fantastic but let me remind you that we're talking about a toxic air pollutant here! How could a toxic free radical, contained within the thick smog spewed from the tailpipe of a gas-guzzling SUV be beneficial for muscle performance and recovery?

The fact that 'increased muscle pump' is a part of that list, alone, should be enough to sound the alarm as to whether or not it's physiologically beneficial. The feeling of inflamed and tight muscles, for which Arnold Schwarzenegger has coined the term "the pump," is caused by increased lactic acid production by cells. Elevating lactic acid levels is the exact opposite of what we want for both muscle performance and good health in general. Lactic acid is well-known to suppress the immune system[9], trigger the release of stress hormones like cortisol[10], reduce carbon dioxide production, causing blood vessels to constrict, and dominantly promotes Cancer growth and metastasis.[11]

I'll discuss nitric oxide's vasodilatory effect shortly, but first, I'd like to shine some light on the impact of misconceptions about nitric oxide on the bodybuilding world. As a result of rigged science by pharmaceutical companies pushing an erection drug through the FDA approval process, we have hundreds, if not thousands, of different allegedly "performance-enhancing" bodybuilding supplements on the market containing the amino acid arginine. Consuming more arginine, whether in the form of food or supplements, like pure arginine powder or high-arginine "superbeet" supplements, will provide the base material from which nitric oxide is synthesized, increasing the amount of nitric oxide produced by your body. Many bodybuilders consume these products believing they're doing themselves a favor and improving their workouts, but unfortunately, they've fallen for a dangerous myth.

Anybody who thinks NO is good for exercise, muscle performance, or sexual function should look at the following study from 2015, which shows that elevated nitric oxide powerfully inhibits testosterone.[12] In the experiment, scientists looked at the effects of nicotine on testosterone levels in male rats. One group of rats received nicotine, and the other received nicotine and a nitric oxide inhibitor called L-NAME. After 30 days of administration, the rats were assessed and their testosterone levels measured. The study showed that testosterone was *significantly decreased* in the group that received the nicotine alone. But in the group that received nicotine as well as the nitric oxide inhibitor, testosterone levels were *significantly higher*. In other words, elevated nitric oxide stimulated by the nicotine decreased testosterone levels. By taking a nitric oxide inhibitor in addition to the nicotine, testosterone levels were maintained.

Another experiment, looking specifically at the effects of nitric oxide on steroidogenesis, came to a similar conclusion.[13] Therefore, if you want your body to produce sufficient testosterone – whether for bodybuilding or general health – it's important you follow these strategies:

- Eat nitrate-free meat.
- Eat vegetables not heavily fertilized with nitrogen.
- Avoid bodybuilding supplements that include nitric oxide precursors like arginine (and erection drugs).

Another nitric oxide precursor that's heavily promoted in the bodybuilding world is the amino acid citrulline. Once ingested, citrulline is sent to the kidneys, where it is converted into the NO precursor arginine, which will then be used to synthesize more NO. And therefore, taking citrulline supplements can cause the same biological calamity as arginine or Viagra by stimulating the production of additional NO.

Viagra: How *Hard* is The Evidence?

Viagra is a drug used to induce erections in men having trouble *getting hard*. This makes for a fun and exciting conversation topic because erections lead to sex, and sex leads to orgasms – and who doesn't love a good orgasm? It is arguably the most pleasurable of all human experiences, at least physically. Taking the drug Viagra is all fun and games, but is it worth losing your life over?

"Warning to Men: Erection Drugs Just Might Kill You" is the title of an article by American author and health journalist Michael Castleman, exposing the potential dangers of Viagra, as well as two other nitric-oxide promoting erection drugs on the market, Cialis and Levitra. Castleman writes:

"The Food and Drug Administration (FDA), the nation's drug-safety watchdog, approved the three main erection drugs as 'safe.' But are they? Not quite. According to a recent study of erection medication side effects during the decade from 1998 (the year Viagra was approved) through 2007, Viagra has been implicated in at least 1,824 deaths mostly from heart attacks. Cialis (approved in 2003) has been linked to 236 deaths, and Levitra (2003) to 121. In addition, the three medications appear to have caused or significantly contributed to at least 2,500 nonfatal heart attacks and other potentially serious heart problems, and more than 25,000 other potentially serious side effects, among them: mini-strokes, vision loss, and hearing loss."

Castleman goes on to expose what he calls the "dirty little secret" of safety studies presented to the FDA, which is that participant pools of men number just a few thousand. "If a drug kills, say, one person in 150,000, that side effect is unlikely to show up during pre-approval trials." The result is that when a drug like Viagra becomes a big seller and is used by millions of men, many of them will drop dead from it.

Soon after Viagra's release in 1998, bodies began dropping like flies. Many of the men who died were getting a double dose of NO by taking Viagra at the same time they were taking the nitrate medication nitroglycerin. We know that nitrates are converted into nitric oxide once inside the body, so the massive spike in funerals that resulted from the co-administration of these two drugs together is a testament to how physiologically devastating nitric oxide can be.

However, what Castleman failed to mention in his article, and is probably not aware of, are the specific consequences of elevating nitric oxide inside the body. It is absolutely essential that Viagra be understood from the perspective of its role as a nitric oxide agonist because it's the precise mechanism by which erection drugs are killing people.

Viagra made nitric oxide famous as the erection chemical, but the list of side effects associated with it make the case for taking it *soft*: Short-term side effects include heart attacks and/or strokes[14]. Chronically elevated nitric oxide long-term causes Cardiovascular Disease,[15] Multiple Sclerosis,[16] Alzheimer's disease, and other types of neurodegenerative dementia.[17] Furthermore, a recent study by scientists at Harvard showed a dramatic increase in the risk of skin Cancer following Viagra use. After following up with over 25,000 men, Viagra users were 84% more likely to develop Melanoma, which is considered the most dangerous of skin cancers.[18]

There's one final and particularly abhorrent potential side effect of Viagra that I feel obligated to tell other men about. In fact, I'd probably grab a ladder, then climb up onto my rooftop and yell this one if I thought it would make a difference.

The Permanent Erection: Gangrene, Impotence & Amputation

It can begin after taking a single dose of Viagra. Just one dose, and after your night of fun, your erection won't go away – for hours, or sometimes even days.[19] Sounds like a dream come true, right? Wrong!

"In some cases, victims have suffered painful erections for several hours and needed hospital treatment. If an erection lasts longer than six hours, it can restrict the blood supply to the intracavernosal smooth muscle in the penis, which facilitates the erection process, causing permanent damage," according to Dr. Roger Kirby, a urologist at St George's Hospital, London.[20] This condition of a prolonged erection is called Priaprism, which is precipitated by a disturbed blood supply departing from the penis to the point where the tissue suffocates, and gangrene of the penis ensues. Penile gangrene is a serious condition in which skin painfully swells and forms blisters that may rupture. Even pus may make an appearance during an episode of penile gangrene.

An article in *Independent* recounts the ghastly experience of a Columbian man who took Viagra to try and impress his girlfriend.[21] The 66-year old Gentil Ramirez Polania popped the erection drug before his big date, and after the party, his erection would not go away. In fact, it lasted several days. When Polania finally went to the hospital complaining of pain, doctors found his penis to be inflamed, *fractured,* and showing signs of gangrene. "In an effort to stop the gangrene from spreading to the rest of the man's body, doctors say they had no option but to remove the man's penis," the article reports.

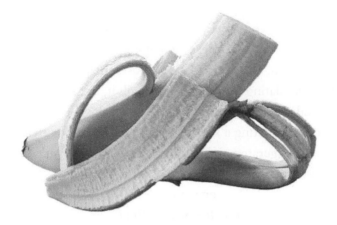

Nitric Oxide and Vasodilation

One of the alleged benefits peddled by proponents of nitric oxide is its vasodilatory effects, meaning it relaxes the inner muscles of the blood vessels, increasing the circulation of blood to tissues of the body that need it. This is the main argument for the theory that nitric oxide supplements are beneficial for the body. However, there is an interesting paradox involved with this phenomenon. In small amounts, the vasodilatory effects of nitric oxide can indeed be beneficial, but what most proponents of nitric oxide supplementation don't realize is that, in excess, it can be causative of a whole host of disorders and pathologies.

If you think of the body mechanically, like a car, which most scientists tend to do, anything that can increase blood vessel dilation will be seen as a good thing. Their thought process goes something like: 'In cardiovascular disease, blood vessels are constricted, so blood vessel constriction *bad!* Nitric oxide causes blood vessels to dilate, so nitric oxide *good!*' An honest misunderstanding of physiology? Mostly. In laboratory experiments, the belief in the dogma that nitric oxide is a miraculous anti-aging molecule is reinforced when scientists observe its immediate vasodilatory effects. But, as previously mentioned, blood vessel dilation isn't always a good thing.

"The idea is that if you increase the diameter of the blood vessels by increasing your nitric oxide, you're going to reverse brain aging by getting more blood circulating. It does help the brain to function by circulating more blood through it, but the problem is that nitric oxide, at the same time, is blocking the ability to use the oxygen, so it's imitating a shock state. In cirrhosis, for example, you get an exaggerated circulation of blood, which isn't being used, because things [like nitric oxide] are inhibiting the oxidative enzymes."

– Dr. Raymond Peat

The paradox of nitric oxide as a vasodilator is that as it causes blood vessels to widen, increasing oxygen transport to areas that were previously hypoxic. It also simultaneously inhibits the capacity of those cells to utilize oxygen. In the exact same way as cyanide or carbon monoxide, nitric oxide "switches off" oxygen use by irreversibly binding directly to the critical respiratory enzyme found within the mitochondria of cells, called cytochrome c oxidase (CCO).[22] CCO is one of the most important metabolic enzymes in the electron transport chain, because it catalyzes the final step in oxidative phosphorylation and interacts directly with oxygen. The result of CCO inhibition by nitric oxide, is reduced energy production by cells.

Constricted blood vessels can undoubtedly be found in people with high blood pressure, and high blood pressure is a precondition for complications like a heart attack or stroke. But when blood vessels are constricted, more nitric oxide isn't the answer. It turns out, nitric oxide is the body's backup mechanism for dilating blood vessels during stress, and the body has its own, much safer way to regulate this process.

Carbon Dioxide: The Body's Primary Vasodilator

"Over the oxygen supply of the body carbon
dioxide spreads its protective wings."
– Professor Johannes Miescher, 1885

Contrary to what nitric oxide enthusiasts believe, the body's primary blood vessel dilator and relaxing factor is not nitric oxide, but another molecule, which does the job far more safely and effectively—carbon dioxide (CO_2). To put it into context, nitric oxide can be thought of as the body's emergency substitute vasodilator when CO_2 is not available.

Students going into the healthcare field are almost universally taught that carbon dioxide is a 'waste product' of cellular metabolism. But far from the waste product, CO_2 is so essential for health that scientist Kyle Mamounis calls it *"the product"* of cellular metabolism. A high concentration of carbon dioxide in the body results in the maintenance of adequate blood vessel dilation and relaxation, and CO_2 is also directly responsible for shuttling oxygen into cells through a phenomenon called *The Bohr Effect.* In one study, intentionally inhaled carbon dioxide was found to reverse pulmonary hypertension induced by oxygen deficiency (hypoxia).[23] In other words, without adequate carbon dioxide, your body cannot use oxygen.

"Do people know that our health depends on
the level of carbon dioxide in the body?"
- Dr. Alina Vasiljeva and Dr. David Nias

One key to understanding carbon dioxide's soothing and calming effect physiologically is that following its production within the mitochondria of cells, it pulls calcium out of the cell and into the bloodstream along with it. This constant streaming of carbon dioxide and removal of calcium from within cells helps balance blood pH and is essential for keeping the "gears" of your body's metabolism "oiled" and efficiently "turning." Nitric oxide and carbon dioxide can both remove calcium from cells, but, unlike CO2, nitric oxide can contribute directly to pathology through its toxicity and inhibitory effects on mitochondrial respiration.

Review   > Mol Cell Biochem. 1997 Sep;174(1-2):189-92.

Nitric oxide inhibition of cytochrome oxidase and mitochondrial respiration: implications for inflammatory, neurodegenerative and ischaemic pathologies

G C Brown [1]

Affiliations + expand
PMID: 9309686

The Nitric Oxide Hypothesis of Aging

One of the most damning studies ever to combat the rolling tidal waves of misinformation regarding nitric oxide is called "The Nitric Oxide Hypothesis of Aging." In the study, scientists from Louisiana State University suggest that nitric oxide is *the primary driver* of aging and causes damage to literally every organ in the body, particularly the brain and heart.

"At the Third International Symposium on the Neurobiology and Neuroendocrinology of Aging, I (McCann, 1997) presented evidence to suggest that excessive production of the free radical, nitric oxide, in the central nervous system and its related glands, such as the pineal and anterior pituitary, may be the most important factor in aging of these structures. Evidence for this hypothesis has been accruing rapidly."

Disease and aging are characterized by the breakdown of efficient cellular energy metabolism inside cells of the body. Nitric oxide's powerful suppressive effects on cellular metabolism explain why it's such a dominant promoter of tissue aging. Russian health researcher Georgi Dinkov describes the transition from health to disease and degeneration from the perspective of nitric oxide:

"Just like the stress hormones, in the short term, NO can be beneficial by preventing direct ischemia [complete loss of oxygen], but when elevated levels of these things become chronic, a general adaptation syndrome begins – a term Hans Selye coined. Then, this biomarker of stress, which was supposed to only be raised short term, becomes raised chronically. Then the body starts to adapt to it and basically, in a state of chronic hypoxia, the body says NO isn't enough, what else should I do to increase blood flow? NO and Lactate are the two most powerful stimulators of angiogenesis – the production of new blood vessels. When you need a wound healed, angiogenesis would be a good thing, but chronically, angiogenesis is one of the primary mechanisms behind the development and spread of Cancer."

If The Nitric Oxide Hypothesis of Aging is correct, reducing nitric oxide in the body is *the most efficient* target to halt aging and degeneration of tissues.

Oh, and by the way, I thought now might be a good time to mention that the caffeine contained in coffee I spoke about at the beginning of this chapter inhibits nitric oxide.[24]

Modern medicine goes astray when it seeks to elevate NO levels until they're contributing directly to pathology. In fact, while the initial effect of nitric oxide may be vasodilation, nitric oxide in excess will quickly cause the opposite to occur, known as vasoconstriction. The following is a perfect (yet tragic) example to illustrate this important point.

Viagra Clinical Trial Kills 11 Babies

Experimenting with Viagra on pregnant women is one of the most shocking and dangerous medical fiascos I've encountered in all my research. Why the f*ck would anyone want to give a pregnant woman the erection drug Viagra!? It turns out, the practice of giving pregnant women the nitric oxide pro-drug Viagra is surprisingly common and approved in most countries for use in an attempt to "improve uteroplacental blood flow, fetal growth, and meaningful infant outcomes."[25] This is a classic example of scientists, who have been taught to view nitric oxide as a vasodilator, thinking more is better. But the tragic results of a 2018 Dutch clinical trial that administered Viagra to pregnant women in an attempt to improve the growth rate of their fetuses have proven otherwise. CNN reports…

"Half of the 183 mothers in the trial had been treated with sildenafil while the other half were treated with a placebo. At the time they were treated, the mothers did not know which treatment they were receiving, which is standard in clinical trials."

"Ninety-three women were treated with the drug, and 90 were treated with the placebo, or dummy pill. Nineteen babies born to the women treated with the drug died, 11 of them due to the lung disorder. Six babies were born with the lung disorder and survived. In comparison, nine babies born to women treated with the placebo died, but none of them had the lung disorder. Three babies with the lung disorder were born to women who were treated with the placebo, and they all survived."

The hope was that the drug would "open up some blood vessels in the placenta," according to Dr. Mohan Pammi, and thereby help the growth of the fetus. But the Dutch researchers found instead that Viagra caused the babies to develop a blood vessel disease in the lungs and increased their risk of death after birth. "The condition is essentially a type of high blood pressure in the lungs [*emphasis added*]," wrote Debra Goldschmidt and Michael Nedelman in the article from CNN. The emphasis I added to the previous quote marks the incredible irony about administering nitric oxide as a vasodilator. Rather than dilating blood vessels, which would lower blood pressure, the initial burst of emergency vasodilation caused by nitric oxide was quickly replaced by vasoconstriction and higher blood pressure, which ended up directly killing the babies.

The Viagra used in the clinical trial was made by the pharmaceutical company Pfizer. Following the study, Pfizer spokeswoman Dervila Keane wrote in an email that the research was "an investigator-initiated study and Pfizer have no involvement in the trial." Keane deflected all questions and responsibility to the scientists involved with the trial.

Perhaps the most shocking and astounding thing about this story is that the use of Viagra on pregnant mothers continues to this day. You'd think that the tragic loss of 11 babies would persuade scientists to halt the use of Viagra on expectant mothers (not to mention question their beliefs about the physiological role of nitric oxide in the body). But instead of admitting nitric oxide is probably not the miracle molecule they've been told, researchers instead blamed the deaths on an incorrect dose and continue their experimentation on pregnant mothers to this day. When will we ever learn!?? Seriously.

Ebola, Bleeding Eyes & Nitric Oxide

In the 1995 blockbuster film *Outbreak*, a fictional town in California is quarantined when it becomes ground zero for an Ebola-like outbreak. The CDC and military medical researchers are tasked with containing and treating infected people who display all the classic symptoms of the Ebola virus, including bleeding from all orifices shortly before dropping dead.

At the end stages of Ebola virus infection, small leaks in blood vessels cause blood to ooze from every hole in the victim's body, followed by a rapid drop in blood pressure that inevitably sends the patient into shock. Immunologist from the University of Texas Thomas Geisbert reports a surprising fact that not many people know: It's not the virus that kills the Ebola patient, but the "cytokine storm" (a signal that causes the immune system to launch its entire arsenal of weapons at once) released by the body's immune system to eliminate the infection that kills the patient.[26] Can you guess the major factor released by the cytokine storm that induces leaky blood vessels and bleeding in Ebola victims?

"Studies show if Ebola patients are going to die, they are very high in nitric oxide, which is what's causing their blood vessels to leak, causing blood to leak out of all their orifices."
– Dr. Raymond Peat

During an outbreak of the Ebola virus in Uganda in 2000, scientists obtained and analyzed blood samples from patients to examine gene expression, antigen levels, and nitric oxide levels. The study found that "blood levels of nitric oxide were much higher in fatal cases (increasing with disease severity)."[27]

If nitric oxide is responsible for the blood-gushing horrors seen in Ebola victims, do you still believe it's a health panacea?

Conclusion

In stark contrast to popular belief and medical dogma, NO is not the miracle molecule it is commonly believed to be. The many tragedies invoked by nitric oxide-promoting drugs like Viagra demonstrate clearly that nitric oxide, in excess, is a destroyer of health and lives.

The colossal and almost universal misunderstanding of nitric oxide in society began when pharmaceutical companies synthesized a drug that they believed would benefit men struggling to get erections. Industry-funded propaganda got the ball rolling on this line of thinking. Then, the reductionist mindset of scientists, which see the body as a machine composed of parts rather than a dynamic living organism, capable of self-regulation, healing, and regeneration, bolstered its momentum to the point where we are at today. Society as a whole now endorses the lie as self-evident.

In isolation, most scientists perceive the observation of blood vessel dilation to be of benefit. But when you zoom out and view the entire organism holistically, it becomes clear that the vasodilator itself can have unfavorable, unintended, and even devastating consequences. Such is the case with the free radical pollutant nitric oxide.

Nitric oxide plays a physiological role in both health and disease, but it is reserved for times of stress. During emergency situations of hypoxia, the body releases nitric oxide to widen blood vessels because if it didn't, the cells would die. But any increase in nitric oxide comes at a price, and that price is a lower metabolic rate through its inhibition of enzymes involved in cellular metabolism.

High levels of nitric oxide in the body are not a marker of health, but rather a marker of damaged, malfunctioning metabolism and aging. Elevating NO chronically through drugs or supplements can accelerate the formation of every known chronic degenerative disease.

So next time you consider popping a Viagra pill or are tempted to purchase NO prodrugs or 'superbeets' loaded with the nitric oxide-precursor arginine to spice up your next workout, I hope you remember this chapter before making a decision. Like the big, bold lettering on the front of a yellow-painted road sign before a treacherous patch of snowy, winding, mountainous road, my suggestion would be, "Proceed with caution."

Key Points to Remember:

- In the 1980s, drug company propaganda convinced the scientific world that nitric oxide was no longer a toxic pollutant, but rather a health-promoting substance to launch their new erection drug Viagra.

- Nitric oxide is a free radical, which means it's highly reactive with other cellular structures, and it tends to increase in the body with age.

- The bodybuilding world has been promoting nitric oxide supplements for decades. Unfortunately, and contrary to what is often claimed by supplement manufacturers, evidence suggests the overall effect of nitric oxide supplementation is reduced testosterone levels, muscle growth, and muscle performance, as well as lower overall health.

- The dangers of elevated nitric oxide are illustrated by looking at the long list of potential side effects associated with nitric oxide-promoting drugs like Viagra, including Heart Attack, Stroke, Cardiovascular Disease, Multiple Sclerosis, Alzheimer's Disease, Dementia, Cancer, and ironically, IMPOTENCE and Penile Gangrene and/or amputation of the penis.

- The body's primary vasodilator is carbon dioxide (CO_2), which is adequately present when cellular metabolism is properly functioning.

- When cellular metabolism isn't working properly, and tissues are deficient in oxygen, the body's backup vasodilator nitric oxide is summoned to combat the hypoxia.

- In small amounts, nitric oxide increases blood flow and provides oxygen to parts of the body that need it.

- In large amounts and/or chronically, nitric oxide has the opposite effect, blocking the body's ability to use oxygen and directly contributing to disease and aging.

- Stress, infection, radiation, and environmental chemicals are all powerful promoters of nitric oxide synthase.

- NO synthesis is part of the body's immune system, produced as a free radical defense mechanism to kill bacteria or other invading microorganisms.

- Nitric oxide induces damage by blocking the essential metabolic enzyme cytochrome c oxidase, which impairs cellular oxygen use.

- Scientists experimenting with Viagra on pregnant women killed 11 babies in 2018. Despite this tragedy, similar experiments continue to this day.

- The blood-leakage from the eyes, ears, mouth and other orifices of the body seen in Ebola patients is caused directly by nitric oxide.

- The Nitric Oxide Hypothesis of Aging suggests nitric oxide is *the primary driver* of aging and causes damage to literally every organ in the body, particularly the brain and heart.

- If The Nitric Oxide Hypothesis of Aging is correct, reducing nitric oxide in the body is *the most efficient* target to halt aging and degeneration of tissues.

- Methylene blue and caffeine are two potent nitric oxide inhibitors.

Gene Therapy Failure
& The Future of Medicine

*"Without self-knowledge, without
understanding the working and functions of his
machine, man cannot be free, he cannot govern
himself and he will always
remain a slave."*
– G. I. Gurdjieff

Mainstream medicine focuses on treating and alleviating symptoms rather than the root cause of disease because it assumes the root cause of disease is something it's not.

The modern medical establishment eagerly funds research aimed at finding genetic causation for disease while snuffing out research intended to reveal disease's true metabolic origins.

Genetic mutations don't cause disease; they are a symptom of mitochondrial dysfunction. Despite the mountain of evidence showing this, which I've documented in my book *Cancer: The Metabolic Disease Unravelled*, the medical industry remains persistent and unwavering in its quest to find solutions for disease in all the wrong places.

The Delusion of Gene Therapy

The future vision of pharmaceutical industrialists is one in which medical treatment is customized for each patient according to their individual genome.[1] They call it "precision medicine," or more commonly, "Gene Therapy" – a paradigm in which drug therapies tailored to the individual are used "to fix broken genes." As exciting and promising as this concept may sound, freelance medical writer and editor of the journal *Biotechnology Healthcare* Jack McCain summed it up when he wrote, "In its current manifestation, gene therapy is an elegant concept crudely executed."[2]

Many people are under the impression that gene therapy's proof-of-concept was demonstrated as early as 1990. Unfortunately, this was due to misinformation and irresponsible reporting by newspapers like the *Los Angeles Times*, claiming Dr. W. French Anderson, "the father of gene therapy," cured a hereditary disease of the immune system in a four-year-old girl.

"That's not quite the way it happened," wrote McCain. It turns out, the purpose of the study had nothing to do with the efficacy of the treatment at all; it was a study simply to test the safety of the treatment. Yes, the patient survived, but what the New York Times article failed to mention was that the patient was treated using conventional therapies before, during, and after gene therapy. To claim that gene therapy was the reason for the patient's survival is a gross misrepresentation of the truth.

Leave it to popular media to twist the truth in favor of the big businesses that fund them. Another thing the article failed to mention was that up until the time of writing, two patients involved in gene therapy trials had died following treatment: one from immune rejection, another from leukemia – in 1999, and 2003, respectively. The entire field of gene therapy, which some believe is 'the holy grail' of medicine, stumbled into existence with false and exaggerated claims.

Theodore Friedmann, MD, who has been deeply involved in the study of gene therapy for many decades (virtually its entire modern history) said the purported success of the initial clinical trial on gene therapy is a "perfect example of the confluence of exaggerated expectations and wishful thinking. Everyone wanted it to work." But, he added, it was unfair to patients and the public that the heightened expectations generated by some of the scientists and their institutions, the media, and others served to raise false hope in many patients with many kinds of disease. "Hope is necessary, but knowingly making undeliverable promises and raising false hope is cruel," Friedmann says. "The delusion of a cure contributed to crashing disappointment later."

"The Father of Gene Therapy" made the following prediction: "Indeed, within 20 years, I expect that gene therapy will be used regularly to ameliorate – and even cure – many ailments." An exciting prospect, indeed. However, he made that prediction in 1995, which means the 20-year window expired many years ago, and today, the routine use of gene therapy is *non-existent*, and nothing even remotely close to a cure has come from it.

As of October 2020, there are eight gene therapy products approved and in clinical use worldwide, including:

1. Gendicine in 2003 in China

2. Glybera in 2012 in Europe

3. Strimvelis in 2016 in Europe

4. Tisagenlecleucel in 2017 in the United States

5. Axicabtagene in 2017 in the United States

6. Luxturna in 2017 in the United States

7. Zolgensma in 2019 in the United States

8. Zynteglo in 2019 in the United States

In stark contrast to Dr. Anderson's predictions about gene therapy, none of the existing approved gene therapies are used regularly, nor are any of them curing people. These therapies are not used regularly because their prices are astronomically high. For example, a single dose of Zolgensma will cost you $2.125 million, officially the most expensive drug of all time.[3] It seems scientists would rather bite their toenails just so their full mouths would give them an excuse not to admit the truth: damaged genes do not cause disease. Yet, despite the monumental failure of gene therapy, the systemic grooming of gene therapy by the media, in bed with the pharmaceutical industry, and by government institutions funding research thus far has remained bulletproof.

"Biomedicine and gene therapies are booming, but we realize, as for other therapeutic approaches, that they suffer intrinsic constraints and limitations and that their most relevant therapeutic fields are complementary to those of traditional drugs. They are now viewed as potentially synergistic with these traditional drugs, rather than competitors," conceded French scientist Jean-Luc Galzi in 2019.[4]

Despite being proven a failure, publishing activity and hope of the "promises" of gene therapy in some scientists somehow remain higher than ever.

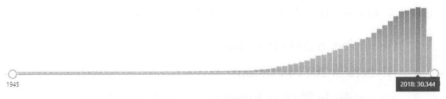

Published papers on gene therapy from 1945-2021

Professor Izpisua Belmonte of the Salk Institute in the US said of gene therapy: "It allows us for the first time to be able to dream of curing diseases that we couldn't before, which is exciting."[5]

Professor Belmonte and scientists who share his excitement can continue dreaming all they want, but the prospect of curing disease using gene therapy will never be anything other than a dream. It's time to leave the genetic-based medical treatment paradigm *in the dust*.

Bioenergetics and the Origins of Frankenstein Cells

"Mitochondrial metabolism is now being seen as the basic
problem in aging and several degenerative diseases."
– Dr. Ray Peat

Anybody who has read my book *Red Light Therapy: Miracle Medicine* knows that the primary mechanism behind red light's remarkable healing potential is its restorative effects on cellular metabolism, specifically through the intensification of the metabolic enzyme cytochrome c oxidase.

Once nitric oxide excesses are dealt with, efficient cellular energy generation resumes, and the body begins using that energy to heal. This mechanism of red light therapy explains the remarkable healing people are experiencing across the world.

Modern scientific research has discovered that basically all known diseases are characterized by widespread dysfunction in metabolism. In other words, if the energy supply of your body is inadequate, your health will suffer. And a lack of health will be accompanied by symptoms, which doctors use to diagnose any number of the 32,000+ officially classified diseases. But regardless of what the symptoms are named, there is only one disease, and the route to recovery is to focus on improving metabolic function within cells.

Vitamins and minerals in the diet provide the raw materials for the production of metabolic enzymes, which is why they're essential. These enzymes can be inhibited by exposure to environmental chemicals. Once nutrient deficiencies and chemical toxicities are addressed, a high metabolic rate can be restored. When it comes to health, *energetics are everything*.

What Causes Genetic Mutations?

DNA strand breaks, genetic mutations, and damage have been demonstrated consistently and repeatedly to be triggered by a condition inside cells known as hypoxia, or insufficient oxygen. In other words, it's the breakdown of mitochondrial function within cells that triggers genetic mutations.

The inhibition of oxygen use by nitric oxide can adequately explain all the horrors associated with the nitric oxide prodrugs like Viagra that you read about in Chapter 1 of this book.

Nitric Oxide > Inhibits CCO > Hypoxia > Genetic Mutations

The downstream consequences of nitric oxide's anti-metabolic effects include genomic instability, genetic errors,[6] double-strand DNA breaks,[7] cell death (apoptosis), inflammation,[8] and ultimately, carcinogenesis.[9] This explains why, after being granted a 'Breakthrough Therapy Designation' by the FDA in 2016 to accelerate the approval process of gene therapy involving the administration of genetically modified T cells, one study reported "No improvement in outcomes with gene therapy for heart failure."[10]

A shoe stuck in the gears of progress

Until people take responsibility for their thoughts and look at the research themselves, like you're doing by reading this book, our tax dollars will continually be funneled into research that will forever result in 'medicine' that prolongs suffering and disease for as long as possible, in an effort to maximize the lifetime profit from each customer. If we want cures or even safe and effective medicines, we must be informed, honest, and bold enough to acknowledge that almost every medicine in the toolbox of a medical doctor will ultimately make our health worse.

Likewise, scientists have struggles of their own that they must acknowledge and find ways to overcome. The gatekeepers of scientific research grants dole out funds for investigations aimed at uncovering genetic causations for disease, while scorning scientists attempting to uncover metabolic origins of disease.

In a plea to fellow scientists and medical professionals, CW Stevens and E Glatstein from the Department of Radiation Oncology at the University of Pennsylvania wrote in a paper called *Beware The Medical-Industrial Complex*:

"We must not be seen as yet another special interest come to drink at the well of public spending, but as advocates for the public good. If we fail to become important to those who control medical spending, we will be unable to make any important long-term contribution to those who matter most – our patients."[11]

The Naked Mole-Rat

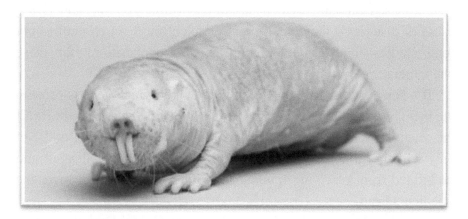

I bet the last thing you expected to see in this chapter was a photo of Dr. Evil's cat. Well not quite. While the skinny, hairless, buck-toothed features of the naked mole-rat may bear a striking resemblance, its remarkable longevity and other features are unique to this fascinating creature.

The naked mole-rat lives its entire life underground in burrows with other rats, spending much of its time tunneling through soil to forage for roots. An article on Endalldisease.com titled *Longevity Secrets of the Naked Mole Rat* reveals many of the robust health qualities of this fascinating creature:

- Naked mole-rats can reproduce from 'puberty' to the grave
- They don't feel pain when being burnt with acid
- They are immune to damage from chemical poisons
- They are immune to Cancer

- They live up to 16x longer than other rats of similar size
- Their tissues *literally* do not age

For decades, scientists have been attempting to explain the extraordinary features of the naked mole-rat but have fallen short. Even in the most recent review, scientists admit they have no idea. The reason for their failure is - in precisely the same fashion that genetic-based human research has failed to discover the underlying cause of diseases – the gatekeepers for scientific research grants only fund studies focusing on finding *genetic* explanations for these phenomena.

If a scientist applies for a grant to discover which gene is causing the increased longevity in the rats, it will probably be approved. But if the scientist wants to study naked mole-rat metabolism, look out! Not only will the grant be rejected, but the threat of being flagged and prohibited from receiving funding for future research looms over the scientist's head.

Friend and independent health researcher Georgi Dinkov emailed one of the scientists working with naked mole-rats asking them to study their metabolism, and he received the following response:

"No way in hell I am going to check metabolism. I got three grants from NIH [The National Institutes of Health] decoding the naked mole-rat genome, so I have no time for this metabolic nonsense."[12]

Can you see a problem with this scientist's approach? Bravo if you said, "Yes, it's unscientific!" The mission of a scientist is to cultivate a high level of critical thinking coupled with a willingness to be wrong about their existing ideas or theories, recognizing that no science is ever entirely settled. Yet, it's clear that this particular scientist's outright and emotionally-charged refusal to question the existing paradigm suggests he is not only failing to embody what it means to be a scientist but has become an impediment to progress and discovery.

Thankfully, not all scientists are that way, and not all scientific research can be controlled. The truth is genetics have *literally nothing* to do with the naked mole-rat's phenomenal health attributes. Scientific findings have revealed to us the fascinating truth: inside naked mole-rat burrows, the composition of the air they breathe is in stark contrast with the atmospheric air of earth.

	Carbon dioxide	Oxygen
Air on Earth	0.04%	20.95%
Mole-Rat Burrow	6.1%	7.2%

By plugging the entrances into their burrows, naked mole-rats modify the oxygen and carbon dioxide content of the air inside, making it ideal for their physiology. Naked mole-rats reduce the oxygen concentration in their burrows to around 7% and increase the CO_2 concentration to around 6%. The result? The increased CO_2 acts as a potent antioxidant while maintaining exceptional blood vessel dilation and cellular oxygenation, resulting in *a very high metabolic rate.* A high metabolic rate can adequately explain all the outstanding physiological features of this charming and handsome subterranean creature.

And if we can humble ourselves and admit that rats are more intelligent than humans, we too can potentially share these same outstanding health features.

One Disease: Mitochondrial Dysfunction

"If we learn to see problems in terms of a general disorder of energy metabolism, we can begin to solve them."
– Dr. Raymond Peat

In The Mitochondrial Theory of Aging, first proposed in 1972,[13] Denham Harman suggests that the rate of aging and onset of disease is determined by the rate of free radical leakage from the electron transport chain inside the mitochondria of cells. Free radicals leak when mitochondrial function fails, and they end up compromising the cell's performance, leading to the traits observed in aging.

The paper *Cellular Metabolism and Disease: What do Metabolic Outliers Teach Us?*[14] gives us an inside look at the revolutionary shift in disease paradigm currently underway, from genetics to metabolism:

"An understanding of metabolic pathways based solely on biochemistry textbooks would underestimate the pervasive role of metabolism in essentially every aspect of biology. It is evident from recent work that many human diseases involve abnormal metabolic states...that perturb normal physiology and lead to severe tissue dysfunction. Understanding these metabolic outliers is now a crucial frontier in disease-oriented research."

Remarkably, this information has been known for literally thousands of years – long before scientists even understood what cellular metabolism was. The scientists wrote:

"This insight predates the formal study of metabolism by many centuries. Almost 2,000 years ago, Celsus knew that rich foods and drink precipitated attacks of gout, and Indian physicians knew that the urine of diabetic patients attracted ants, whereas normal urine did not. A greater appreciation for the relationship between precise metabolic activities and disease states blossomed during the golden age, but momentum in metabolic research gradually dissipated with the advent of newer areas of biological investigation in the latter half of the 20th century and perhaps from the suspicion that most of what could be known about intermediary metabolism had already been discovered. The search for the genetic and molecular bases of Cancer, diabetes, obesity, and neurodegeneration displaced focus from understanding the altered metabolic states in these diseases. Many common diseases are now understood in terms of inherited or somatic mutations that impact gene expression, signal transduction, cellular differentiation, and other processes not traditionally viewed in bioenergetic or metabolic terms."

Here we are in the 21st century, and progress from modern science has actually brought us back in time to the truth that was once known, yet forgotten.

Powerful economic forces grip tightly onto the highly profitable yet utterly failed paradigm of genetic causation of disease. But the truth has torn through the fabric of that paradigm, and there is no needle and thread in existence that can repair it. Pandora's box has been opened, and never again can it be sealed.

The Rise of Metabolic Therapies

Therapies that target cellular metabolism for repair are the final frontier in medicine. Nutrients, therapies, and drugs that effectively enhance the body's metabolic rate already exist on the market today. And miraculously, some of the finest medicines are also the least expensive, most easily obtainable, and come with virtually no side effects.

If we consciously seek out and utilize only remedies that target metabolic deficiency, while avoiding toxic drugs that target symptoms, we can thrive, not just survive, the great transition from genetic to metabolic medicine.

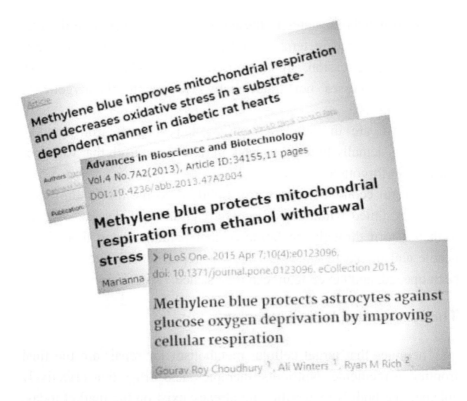

Methylene blue improves mitochondrial respiration and decreases oxidative stress in a substrate-dependent manner in diabetic rat hearts

Advances in Bioscience and Biotechnology
Vol.4 No.7A2(2013), Article ID:34155,11 pages
DOI:10.4236/abb.2013.47A2004

Methylene blue protects mitochondrial respiration from ethanol withdrawal stress

> PLoS One. 2015 Apr 7;10(4):e0123096.
doi: 10.1371/journal.pone.0123096. eCollection 2015.

Methylene blue protects astrocytes against glucose oxygen deprivation by improving cellular respiration

Gourav Roy Choudhury [1], Ali Winters [1], Ryan M Rich [2]

Key Points to Remember:

- Genetic mutations don't cause disease; they are a symptom of Mitochondrial Dysfunction.

- Propaganda has convinced many scientists that gene therapy is 'the holy grail' of medicine.

- Gene therapy has been a complete and utter failure; it has provided no meaningful treatments, let alone cures.

- Naked mole-rats are immune to Cancer, and their tissues literally do not age due to their extraordinarily high metabolic rates.

- The metabolic origins of disease have been known for almost 2000 years, long before metabolism was studied scientifically.

- Modern scientific breakthroughs have brought us *back* in time to the truth that was once known yet forgotten.

- Only one disease exists: Metabolic Dysfunction.

- Therapies that target the metabolism for repair are the final frontier in medicine.

- Some of the finest metabolic medicines are also the safest and least expensive.

- Methylene blue might be the most potent metabolic therapy ever discovered.

PART II:
Methylene Blue

—

The Great Nitric Oxide Inhibitor

Meet Methylene Blue

Methylene blue (methylthioninium chloride) is one of the oldest organic dyes ever produced. In 1876, German chemist Heinrich Caro, head of research at the world's largest chemical producing company BASF, first synthesized this pure blue dye to stain wool for the textile industry. But it wasn't long before medical researchers discovered uses for methylene blue far beyond fabric coloring. The vast and expansive utility of methylene blue suddenly bled from the fabric industry into medicine.

In 1880, microbiologist Robert Koch pioneered the use of methylene blue for staining cells and microbes for easier visualization under a microscope. As a stain in microscopy, methylene blue can help scientists distinguish dead cells from living cells. It can also help them study the internal components of cells by highlighting their anatomical structures. Koch began using methylene blue to stain tuberculosis-causing bacteria to better understand Tuberculosis,[1] and Polish pathologist Czeslaw Checinski used it to stain Malaria-causing parasites to better understand Malaria. Not only is methylene blue capable of staining the Malaria-causing parasite, but it was found also to be capable of killing it, noted German physician and Nobel Prize laureate Paul Ehrlich.[2] In 1891, Ehrlich published a case study on two Malaria patients who were allegedly cured using methylene blue.[3] Its use for the treatment of Malaria awarded methylene blue the honor of being the first pharmaceutical drug in history.

During the Second World War, methylene blue was given to soldiers as an antimalarial drug.[4] Their blue-colored urine was found useful for doctors as a means to know whether or not they were adhering to their methylene blue drug treatment regimens.[5]

Complaints from WWII soldiers and patients about methylene blue coloring their urine blue soon stimulated a transition to other drugs to treat Malaria. However, modern research has revived interest in using methylene blue as an antimalarial, and it is considered one of the most, if not the most, effective drug for the disease to this day.[6]

Methylene Blue and The Brain

While studying methylene blue in his lab, Ehrlich observed that it would quickly concentrate in the brain once injected into animals. This gives the drug enormous potential for conditions involving the brain, which we will explore in greater detail in upcoming chapters.

Methylene blue was one of the first drugs used to treat patients with psychosis at the end of the 19th century. It was studied for bipolar disorder in the 1980s. Since then, it has been under investigation for its potential use in dementia and other neurodegenerative related disorders.[7]

Methylene Blue Targets Diseased Tissues

Methylene blue's uncanny ability to selectively target diseased tissues in the body was another observation made by Ehrlich. Although healthy tissues could benefit from the methylene blue, the cells with the greatest dysfunction metabolically received aid first. Inspired by his research into methylene blue, Ehrlich coined the term "magic bullet," which is still in use today.

Methylene Blue Redox Test for Milk

In the 1940s and 1950s, the methylene blue redox test was used to determine the freshness of milk by indirectly revealing how much oxygen is inside the milk.

Add a couple of drops of methylene blue to a glass of milk, and the methylene blue will slowly decolorize in proportion to the amount of oxygen in it. The less oxygen (the closer to spoiled), the more quickly the blue color will disappear.

Although, in a sense, milk never *really* spoils; it ferments into other delicious and nourishing products like yogurt and cheese. People buying milk generally want it fresh and unfermented. So in this context, it is considered spoiled when oxygen is used up, and living cells within it are then forced to begin producing energy fermentatively (without oxygen) as opposed to oxidatively (with oxygen).

"The methylene blue reduction test is as accurate a measure of the keeping quality of milk as any method yet available. It will divide milks into three or four classes with reasonable accuracy, as will any of a number of tests for milk quality. It is inexpensive and as nearly fool-proof as any method for this purpose available to the dairy bacteriologist."[8]
– Thornton, 1930

Methylene Blue Redox Skin Test

Similar to the milk test, if you put a drop of methylene blue on your skin, the quicker it disappears, the more starved for oxygen (hypoxic) that local tissue is. Since methylene blue substitutes for oxygen, the more hypoxic the skin tissue, the quicker it gets used.

According to independent health researcher Gyorgyi Dinkov, if the methylene blue drop on your skin completely disappears in less than six hours, it indicates local hypoxia.

How Methylene Blue Works

The trillions of cells of which your body is comprised are the foundations of life itself. It's the mitochondria within your cells that produce the biological energy in the form of a molecule called ATP, the "energy currency" of the body. Any increase in ATP production will be beneficial, particularly to individuals who are sick.

Research into the therapeutic value of methylene blue dates back to the 1800's, but only within the past couple of decades have scientists decoded exactly how methylene blue provides its benefits to the brain and body, spanning all the way down to the molecular level in the mitochondria.

Methylene blue works by directly increasing mitochondrial respiration through its interactions with the electron transport chain. The electron transport chain is a series of four protein complexes that sit inside the mitochondrial membrane and are responsible for producing ATP—a process called oxidative phosphorylation. The remarkable therapeutic effects of methylene blue are predicated by its ability to act as an alternative electron carrier when any of the mitochondrial complexes I-IV are dysfunctional.

The primary ways that methylene blue benefits the body is its role as a nitric oxide inhibitor and an estrogen antagonist. By reducing nitric oxide and estrogen, thyroid function is increased, and the body benefits from increased metabolic rate and overall energy production. Below is a list of the ways methylene blue improves metabolism.

3 Ways Methylene Blue Inhibits Nitric Oxide

- Inhibits nitric oxide synthesis[9]
- Disassociates nitric oxide from cytochrome c oxidase enzyme[10]
- Scavenges existing nitric oxide[11] [12]

Methylene Blue Effects on Metabolism

- Increases oxygen consumption and ATP production[13]
- Increases glucose consumption[14]
- Increases the NAD/NADH ratio[15]
- Decreases lactic acid production[16]

- Is a potent antioxidant; acts similarly to vitamin E[17]
- Inhibits monoamine oxidase (MAO)[18]
- Acts as an alternative electron carrier in the mitochondrial electron transport chain[19]

Methylene Blue Effects on Hormones

- Inhibits prolactin[20]
- Inhibits estrogen[21]
- Increases thyroid hormone and lowers TSH[22][23]
- Increases testosterone[24]

Modern interest in Methylene Blue Skyrocketing

In recent years, research into the use of methylene blue has skyrocketed. Never in history has there been more interest and scientific papers published involving methylene blue.

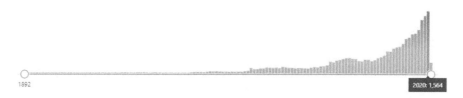

1892   2020: 1,564

Published papers on methylene blue from 1892-2021

As the research train rolls on, scientists discover more and more uses for methylene blue that can benefit many disease pathologies safely and effectively.

The world is catching on to the fact that all diseases are metabolic in nature, and that methylene blue selectively targets cells and tissues that have dysfunctional metabolism. It's only a matter of time before methylene blue is recognized as one of the most potent medicines ever discovered.

Top 10 Benefits of Methylene Blue

Now that you've been acquainted with methylene blue, it's time to discover some of the remarkable things methylene blue can do for your health by diving straight into the scientific and clinical research. This information is probably why you purchased this book in the first place, so I'm glad you've made it this far.

Here's my official list of the top 10 benefits of methylene blue.

1. An Antidote for Chemical Poisoning and Overdose
2. The Greatest Anti-Malarial Drug Ever Discovered?
3. Methylene Blue: The Virus Warrior
4. Forget Dementia: MB for Alzheimer's and Parkinson's
5. Cognitive Enhancement: A Brain-Boosting Powerhouse
6. Depression No More
7. Hope for Autism?
8. The Great Pain Reliever
9. A Healthier Heart
10. Methylene Blue vs. Cancer

1. An Antidote for Chemical Poisoning and Overdose

If you thought methylene blue was some obscure and occult medicinal chemical that's not well known or is not yet in widespread use in this world, think again. "MB [methylene blue] is always present as the main antidote required in emergency and critical care units," wrote a group of scientists in a scientific review article published in 2018.[1] In fact, methylene blue is so essential and routinely used in hospital emergency rooms that scientists from the United States, Japan, Greece, Italy, and Canada have stressed the importance of stockpiling it. Situations in which methylene blue is routinely used in hospital emergency rooms include circulatory shock, neuroprotection, anaphylaxis (severe allergic reactions), and overdoses and chemical poisonings.

Around 1930, Matilda Moldenhauer Brooks, Ph.D. suggested using methylene as an antidote for cyanide and carbon monoxide poisoning, which stemmed from a number of studies she conducted on animals.[2] Since then, cyanide victims in critical care units worldwide have been treated successfully using methylene blue. But methylene blue works as an antidote for far more than just cyanide and carbon monoxide poisoning.

It's important to understand that chemical poisonings induce a situation in the body called methemoglobinemia, which is the one and only condition methylene blue has been FDA approved to treat. Once you understand this condition and how methylene blue can remedy it, you'll comprehend its value as an antidote for virtually all chemical poisonings and why hospital emergency rooms commonly use it for this application.

Methemoglobinemia is a blood disorder that occurs when hemoglobin, contained inside red blood cells, becomes oxidized and loses its capacity to transport oxygen. The oxidized form of hemoglobin is called methemoglobin, hence the name methemoglobinemia. The presence of high levels of methemoglobin in the blood leads to tissue hypoxia. Without oxygen, nitric oxide and a cascade of stress hormones and pro-inflammatory signals are all increased, and the body's energy supply is essentially switched *off*.

Symptoms of Methemoglobinemia

Common symptoms of methemoglobinemia include blue fingertips (cyanosis), shortness of breath (dyspnea), confusion, seizures, coma, and metabolic acidosis. Chocolate brown-colored blood is another one of the definitive characteristics of methemoglobinemia.

Causes of Methemoglobinemia

- Cyanide

- Carbon monoxide

- Sodium nitrite/nitrate

- Acetaminophen

- Formaldehyde

- Pharmaceutical drugs

- The party drug 'poppers' (amyl nitrate)

- Lidocaine, benzocaine and other anesthetics

- Heavy metals like aluminum, copper, cadmium, etc.

- Fluoride, found in toothpaste

- Chlorine dioxide-based household cleaning products

- Chemicals found in drugstore shampoos, deodorants and soaps

- COVID-19 can also induce methemoglobinemia

Methylene Blue Treatment for Methemoglobinemia

When emergency room patients with methemoglobinemia are treated using methylene blue, it acts as a potent antidote by converting methemoglobin back to hemoglobin, restoring its oxygen-carrying capacity. Then, oxygen can be transported throughout the body to the cells and tissues where it is needed. Once oxygen use is restored, all the symptoms experienced by the patient are then resolved.

Most medical personnel administering methylene blue for chemical poisonings and overdoses are not aware that methylene blue's value as an antidote extends far beyond its capacity to convert oxidized hemoglobin back to its regular form. In a 2018 study examining the use of methylene blue for cyanide poisoning, scientists wrote: "Its protective effects appear to be related to the unique properties of this redox dye, which, depending on the dose, could directly oppose some of the consequences of the metabolic depression produced by CN [cyanide] at the cellular level." In other words, methylene blue corrected the defective cellular metabolism caused by the poison.[3]

2. The Greatest Anti-Malarial Drug Ever Discovered?

"Even at the loo, we see, we pee, navy blue," observed soldiers given methylene blue during World War II. Allied forces in the South Pacific widely used Methylene blue to prevent and treat Malaria infection during the second world war.[4] Despite it keeping them healthy and being well-tolerated, most soldiers didn't like it because it caused blue-colored urine.

Prior to methylene blue, the classic treatment for Malaria was a compound called quinine, which is an alkaloid contained within the bark of a cinchona tree native to South America. The bark of the cinchona tree was first employed to treat Malaria in Europe during the 15th century.[5] Interestingly, the carbonated beverage known as tonic water contains quinine, which some people drink to ease leg cramps. If you can handle the bittersweet tang of tonic water, between the quinine, glucose, and the carbon dioxide contained within it, you've got yourself a refreshing and medicinal beverage.

Following the discovery and synthesis of methylene blue, suddenly Malaria medicine could be produced on a large scale in a laboratory, without needing to be laboriously isolated from a plant bark only available in South America. This represented a quantum leap in Malaria treatment and medicine.

But since methylene blue stains the mouth and tends to color urine bluish-green, scientists began altering the molecular structure of methylene blue, attempting to remove the tint while maintaining its medicinal qualities. The work of chemists like Wilhelm Rohl of Bayer, a student of Ehrlich's, eventually gave rise to the drug quinacrine for Malaria. Then in 1934, quinacrine was modified by Hans Andersag of Bayer, which resulted in the synthesis of chloroquine, used as the standard treatment for Malaria to this day.[6]

You may have heard doctors talk about the use of hydroxychloroquine as an effective antidote to the 2020 viral pandemic COVID-19. It turns out that hydroxychloroquine is derived from methylene blue; methylene blue is its parent compound, which reveals methylene blue's potential for treating COVID and other viruses, a subject we will soon explore.

One of the challenges with Malaria treatment is that Malarial parasites, such as Plasmodium falciparum, show increased resistance to common antimalarial drugs. This has prompted scientists like Professor Olaf Müller of Heidelberg University to revisit using methylene blue as an antimalarial.[7] Cell culture experiments show that methylene blue has remarkable antimalarial potency at very low doses. Perhaps most importantly, experiments show that resistance to methylene blue is also very low.[8]

The new generation of methylene blue research as an antimalarial agent has proven that no drug even comes close to the potency or effectiveness of methylene blue against Malaria. Dr. Ehrlich reported in 1891 to have completely cured two Malaria patients using methylene blue.[9] Similarly, scientists from Radboud University Medical Center in the Netherlands reported in 2018 to have also completely cured Malaria patients using methylene blue *in just 48 hours.*[10] This was an unprecedented rate – far quicker than any other known drug or remedy. Additionally, patients no longer transmitted the parasite when they were bitten by a mosquito following treatment.

"Methylene blue is very promising, because it can prevent the spread of Malaria within such a short time following treatment. There are also indications that methylene blue also works well in species that are resistant to certain medicines."

– Teun Bousema, study coordinator

It appears that all the "advancements" in new generations of antimalarial drugs since methylene blue were not advancements at all and methylene blue is still the victor.

On World Malaria Day in 2018, German researchers published a meta-analysis on the use of methylene blue for Malaria and concluded it is highly effective against the Malaria-causing parasite in all endemic areas.[11]

3. Methylene Blue: The Virus Warrior

The life cycles of parasites, bacteria, fungi, and viruses are all in jeopardy when in the presence of methylene blue. And when used in combination with light therapy, methylene blue exerts even greater antimicrobial effects against bacteria, like E. coli and others[12], including drug-resistant strains,[13] against fungi like candida,[14] and also against many common viruses, including Zika, West Nile, Ebola, Hepatitis, and HIV.

"If a fart can go through your underwear,
a virus can go through a mask."
– My 5-year-old nephew

After the COVID-19 pandemic was declared in spring 2020, my nephew's words brought my family and me some much-needed laughter.

Regardless of your take on the use of masks, forced isolation, or your government's response to the COVID-19 pandemic, one thing we can all agree on is it would be nice to have a way to effectively prevent and eliminate viruses, so we never have to ride the turbulent wake of a pandemic again.

Methylene Blue Terminates COVID, HIV, Ebola, Zika and Other Viruses

The value of methylene blue as an antiviral has a rich history in the scientific literature. It has proven itself valuable against many of the viruses considered to be serious threats to humanity. Methylene blue might be the greatest antiviral that will ever be, not only for the virus responsible for COVID-19, but also for many other popular and allegedly dangerous viruses. What's more, when you combine light therapy with methylene blue, these two powerful mitochondrial therapies synergize together and result in significantly enhanced antiviral activity.

Here are some examples of antiviral activity methylene blue has shown alone and in combination with light therapy. When used with light therapy, the treatment is called photodynamic therapy, which you'll soon learn more about for various diseases.

- Methylene blue inactivates Zika virus & Sindbis virus[15]

- Methylene blue + light inactivates West Nile virus[16]

- Methylene blue + light reduces Ebola virus infectivity

- Methylene blue + light reduces Middle East respiratory syndrome virus infectivity[17]

- Methylene blue + light reduces HIV-1 "to nondetectable levels"

- Methylene blue + light reduces Bovine Diarrhea virus "to nondetectable levels"

- Methylene blue + light reduces Pseudorabies virus "to nondetectable levels"

- Methylene blue + light reduces Hepatitis A virus

- Methylene blue + light reduces Porcine Parvovirus[18]

- Methylene blue + light inactivates Enterovirus 71[19]

- Methylene blue + light inactivates Flavivirus[20]

- Methylene blue + light inactivates Herpes virus[21]

- Methylene blue + light inactivates Dengue virus[22]

Methylene Blue for COVID-19

The virus responsible for the COVID-19 pandemic (SARS-CoV-2) has affected our lives profoundly and in some ways permanently. Did you ever think you'd be living in a world where people were afraid to shake hands, hug, or even be near someone?

Almost immediately following the declaration of the COVID-19 pandemic by the World Health Organization in March 2020, behind the scenes, scientists from across the world got to work searching for ways to inhibit the replication and spread of the virus. Chinese scientists were among the first to investigate methylene blue's effects on COVID-19. In March 2020, they published a study reporting methylene blue can "effectively eliminate SARS-CoV-2 in vitro within two minutes [*emphasis added*].[23]" Two minutes!? Why didn't the public hear about this?

It took quite a long time before scientists in other countries followed up on these findings. In October 2020, French researchers duplicated the study in their lab and came to the same conclusion: In very low doses, methylene blue possesses powerful antiviral activity against SARS-CoV-2. Their study concluded, "We propose that methylene blue is a promising drug for the treatment of COVID-19."[24]

Doctor Claims Methylene Blue Derivative Cures COVID-19

You may have seen the viral [no pun intended] video of Nigerian doctor Stella Immanuel, claiming she used hydroxychloroquine to cure hundreds of COVID patients, which was quickly censored and pulled from social media websites. (Why did they pull it?) It turns out, this effective drug against COVID is actually derived *from* methylene blue. In other words, methylene blue is a parent compound of the hydroxychloroquine that is to this day the primary treatment for Malaria and found to be effective, and some say curative, against COVID-19.

Can Methylene Blue Block COVID Transmission?

Cancer patients have a higher-than-normal risk of viral infection due to compromised immune systems and overall poor health status. When scientists administered methylene blue to 2500 Cancer patients, none of them ended up developing COVID-19.[25] Coincidence? Or is methylene blue a first-class preventative?

How COVID Manifests in the Body

It's important to understand how COVID-19 affects the body. The way it manifests is something you are now familiar with if you've read the preceding chapters in this book. A study from January 2021 showed that COVID is simply another case of widespread mitochondrial dysfunction.[26] Its pathology is exactly the same as virtually all other diseases, including Diabetes, Cancer, Heart Disease, Obesity, Alzheimer's, etc.

"We demonstrate mitochondrial dysfunction, metabolic alterations with an increase in glycolysis… from patients with COVID-19… These data suggest that patients with COVID-19 have a compromised mitochondrial function and an energy deficit that is compensated by a metabolic switch to glycolysis. This metabolic manipulation by SARS-CoV-2 triggers an enhanced inflammatory response that contributes to the severity of symptoms in COVID-19," wrote scientists from Kings College Hospital in London, UK and The University of Alabama at Birmingham.[27]

What that means is COVID inhibits cellular metabolism, and methylene blue works by powerfully restoring metabolic function to cells.

Scientists Testing Nitric Oxide to Treat COVID-19?

I want to address the recent flood of research reporting that nitric oxide can inhibit the replication of COVID-19, which is another fantastic example of mass ignorance within the scientific community. Yes, choking off the energy supply of an infected cell in a petri dish by poisoning it with a free radical like nitric oxide will inhibit its ability to create the proteins necessary for viral replication. But due to the reductionist mindset and lack of understanding of how the body actually works, these scientists fail to recognize the overwhelmingly negative consequences of introducing a dose of toxic free radicals into a living organism.

As we've explored thoroughly in previous chapters, nitric oxide forcefully damages cellular mitochondrial function and metabolic activity within all cells of the body. Likewise, one of the primary reasons methylene blue is so effective against viruses is that it *reduces* nitric oxide levels, which upregulates energy availability, enhancing the body's innate immune defenses, helping it abolish the virus on its own.

A 2021 review of Methylene blue for COVID-19 reports:

"The only drug known to inhibit the excessive production of reactive species and cytokines is methylene blue, a low-cost dye with antiseptic properties used effectively to treat Malaria, urinary tract infections, septic shock, and methemoglobinaemia."[28]

---

4. Forget Dementia: MB vs Alzheimer's and Parkinson's

The CDC, Mayo clinic, and other pop culture health pundits admit they have no idea what causes Alzheimer's and other forms of dementia. For around 50 years, they have focused funding on genetic research, believing that genetic defects cause Alzheimer's, but the genetic theory has never been proven. As a result of their commitment to genetic causation, they ignore the trail of evidence leading to the true cause of dementia. Let's dust off that trail now and shine a spotlight on the evidence.

A groundbreaking study from 2017 reports that as the brain ages, mitochondrial metabolism decreases and that this phenomenon is possibly the *main culprit* behind many neurological diseases, including Alzheimer's and Parkinson's.[29] If your brain has sufficient energy, it will function effectively – from memory retrieval speed, concentration, and focus, etc. As the metabolic rate of the brain declines with age, so too does your ability to think, remember, and speak clearly.

In recent years, the role of nitric oxide (NO) in the formation and progression of dementia-related disorders like Alzheimer's disease has come to light. For example, NO has been found to accumulate around the plaques inside the brain of Alzheimer's patients,[30] and it's also been hypothesized that NO could be responsible for brain cell death found in Alzheimer's and other forms of dementia.[31] All of these suggest that using a nitric oxide inhibitor such as methylene blue could be a remarkably effective tool for dealing with dementia.

One fascinating and useful attribute of methylene blue for treating brain disorders is that, once inside the body, it tends to accumulate in the brain, right where it is needed. This makes its potential as a therapy of particular interest for dementia and all kinds of brain-related disorders.

The Acetylcholine Myth

If current medical drugs prescribed to Alzheimer's patients worked, then the disease would no longer exist. But the disease *does* exist – and its prevalence is higher than ever before in history and is expected to increase going forward. I've included this section on the role of acetylcholine in Alzheimer's and brain aging to clear up some misconceptions and explain why medical doctors have neither the tools nor the knowledge to help someone with this condition. Dr. Ray Peat explains...

"The current popular medical approach to treating Alzheimer's disease is to try and increase the level of acetylcholine by blocking the enzyme that breaks it down. And they've demonstrated that it doesn't work, and so they need a new fundamental theory, but their theory is so mistaken it's hard for them to get off onto a new line of drug treatment.

Acetylcholine is essential and part of our conscious regulation and all kinds of biological processes, but it activates the enzyme that produces nitric oxide and nitric oxide blocks energy production. And so, the process of excitotoxicity that made monosodium glutamate notorious, because a little too much of it activates the production of a little too much acetylcholine, which makes too much nitric oxide.

Nitric oxide poisons the ability to oxidize glucose into carbon dioxide, increases lactic acid, and the cell has less energy and is more excited by the acetylcholine, so basically it becomes susceptible to dying in proportion to the overstimulation of acetylcholine."

- Dr. Ray Peat

Once again, the reality turns out to be exactly the opposite of what the for-profit mainstream medical industry claims. Acetylcholine *accumulates* as both brain and body age, so taking drugs to increase acetylcholine even more, which medical doctors will prescribe, can only make the situation worse.

The rational approach to treating Alzheimer's disease is to *decrease* the production and action of acetylcholine in the brain. Listed below is some of the existing scientific evidence in support of the idea that too much acetylcholine can have negative effects on the health of the brain and body:

- During slow-wave sleep (SWS), low acetylcholine levels in the hippocampus are essential for long-term storage of declarative memories to occur. Studies have shown that increasing acetylcholine during SWS "completely blocked SWS-related consolidation of declarative memories for word pairs in human subjects."[32]

- Drugs that block acetylcholine production (by blocking nicotinic acetylcholine receptors) have anti-depressant-like effects in animal studies.[33] [34]

- People with hives tend to have higher acetylcholine in their skin, which causes excess histamine to be produced and reduces sweating. Drugs that block acetylcholine are being investigated for preventing hive outbreaks.[35] [36]

How to Reduce Acetylcholine

There are two approaches to lowering acetylcholine. First, inhibit acetylcholine production by blocking acetylcholine receptors. Second, increase cholinesterase, the enzyme that breaks down acetylcholine.

1. **How to reduce acetylcholine production** – Methylene blue reduces acetylcholine production by blocking acetylcholine receptors.[37]
2. **How to increase acetylcholine breakdown** – "A rich environment increases the enzyme that breaks down acetylcholine," said Dr. Peat, which includes "having lots of fun, reading interesting things, and talking to interesting people."

Can Methylene Blue Cure Dementia?

In 2019, scientists gave Alzheimer's patients 8mg-16mg of methylene blue daily while monitoring their brain function. They witnessed the methylene blue treatment stop Alzheimer's disease dead in its tracks.[38] [39]

"Treatment with 8mg-16mg MB daily reduced cognitive decline by more than 85%! That is the perverted medical profession's way of saying that MB effectively stopped AD in its tracks, or at least its cognitive symptoms, which is what this disease is all about. It is a type of dementia after all. Perhaps just as importantly, it found that drugs currently approved for managing symptoms of AD interfere with the therapeutic benefit of MB when administered together with it!"
– Georgi Dinkov

When a therapy stops cognitive decline by 85% over 65 weeks, as it did in the study, at what point do we say it cured the patient? If your answer is 100%, then perhaps methylene blue is about as close to a cure as it gets.

Treatment Dose for Dementia

For those interested in using methylene blue for Alzheimer's, an important finding from the study was that a dose of 200mg of methylene blue had *no greater benefit* than a much smaller dose of 8mg. The study concluded that methylene blue is expected to be therapeutic in doses up to 16mg, and patients would see no additional benefit from taking higher doses. "Treatment benefit is predicted to be maximal at 16mg/day as monotherapy," the scientists reported.

Methylene Blue and The Hallmarks of Alzheimer's Disease

Scientists studying the brains of Alzheimer's patients noticed a few things that are common or universal among patients, which they refer to as hallmarks of the disease. One hallmark of neurodegeneration is abnormally shaped tau proteins, or "neurofibrillary tangles" within brain cells called neurons.

Hallmark 1: Neurofibrillary "Tangles"

When mice are genetically engineered to lack tau protein, their brain cells do not function properly, leading researchers to believe that the misshapen tau proteins found in brain cells of Alzheimer's patients play a role in the disease. Soeda, Saito, Maeda, Nakamura, Kojima, and Takashima, a team of scientists from Gakushuin University and Keio University School of Medicine in Japan, published a study in 2019 that reports methylene blue can fix this issue by inhibiting the formation of tau neurofibrillary tangles in the brain.[40]

Hallmark 2: Beta Amyloid Plaques

Another classic hallmark of the Alzheimer's brain is the presence of beta amyloid plaques surrounding brain cells. Remarkably, methylene blue has been shown scientifically to prevent beta amyloid plaques from forming on the outside of neurons.[41]

As you've seen in this section, evidence suggests the resolution of both of the hallmarks of Alzheimer's disease using methylene blue. Not bad for a fabric dye.

Lies and Manipulation by Big Pharma

In July 2016, mainstream media outlets reported that a patented form of methylene blue called LMTX, developed by TauRx Pharmaceuticals, "failed to improve cognitive and functional skills in patients with mild to moderate Alzheimer's disease."[42] But wait! A closer look at the clinical trial reveals methylene blue only failed when combined with highly excitotoxic drugs currently used for the treatment of Alzheimer's disease. In patients that took methylene blue on its own, the therapy worked.

"...But in a perplexing twist, the drug did show a significant benefit in about 15 percent of patients in the trial who were not taking other standard Alzheimer's drugs, according to the findings released on Wednesday at the Alzheimer's Association International Conference in Toronto." In a classic manipulative strategy by pharmaceutical companies, a dose of poison was given to patients along with methylene blue to make it appear ineffective, thus killing the incentive for further research.

In November 2017, results from a second phase III study were published, showing once again benefits of methylene blue as a monotherapy. Attempts to thwart research into methylene blue appear to have been averted by scientists, who concluded, "In order to get a clearer idea of the effects of LMTX, we now need to see carefully planned studies that focus on LMTX alone and don't involve people who are taking other Alzheimer's medications."[43] The research continues.

The *Metabolic* Hallmarks of Alzheimer's Disease

As you've deduced from reading this chapter, the details of dementia can be infinitely complex. Still, the truth can also be made simple by realizing that the decline in mitochondrial metabolism is what neurological diseases like Alzheimer's and Parkinson's are all about. We've gone over some of the hallmarks of Alzheimer's disease purported by mainstream sources, but it's evident that the aggregation of beta amyloid plaques and neurofibrillary tangles are likely *effects* rather than causes. The plaques and tangles are downstream epiphenomenon occurring after the breakdown of efficient cellular metabolism.

I've taken the liberty to create a description of two *metabolic* hallmarks of dementia below, which appear to far more accurately represent the physiological conditions causative of dementia and other forms of neurodegeneration.

Hallmark 1: Decreased Mitochondrial Complex IV Function

In Alzheimer's, one of the specific metabolic hallmarks is a decline in complex IV function within the mitochondria of cells. Complex IV of the electron transport chain involves the enzyme cytochrome c oxidase, which interacts directly with oxygen and catalyzes the final step in cellular respiration. It turns out methylene blue has a restorative effect on complex IV.

A 2007 animal experiment administered methylene blue (1mg/kg) to rats once a day for three days and found that brain cytochrome c oxidase activity was 70% higher than in the placebo-treated group.[44] The improved memory consolidation that resulted from the methylene blue treatment was attributed to the increase in metabolic activity of the brain.

In 2008, researchers from the Nutrition & Metabolism Centre at Children's Hospital Oakland Research Institute in California reported that methylene blue extends the lifespan of human cells by enhancing mitochondrial function, specifically complex IV activity. "MB increases mitochondrial complex IV by 30%, enhances cellular oxygen consumption by 37-70%, increases heme synthesis, and reverses premature senescence [aging]."[45]

"The results are very encouraging," said Dr. Atamna, the study's lead author. "We'd eventually like to try to prevent the physical and cognitive decline associated with aging, with a focus on people with Alzheimer's disease. One of the key aspects of Alzheimer's disease is mitochondrial dysfunction, specifically complex IV dysfunction, which methylene blue improves. Our findings indicate that methylene blue, by enhancing mitochondrial function, expands the mitochondrial reserve of the brain. Adequate mitochondrial reserve is essential for preventing age-related disorders such as Alzheimer's disease."

"What we potentially have is a wonder drug." said Dr. Ames. "To find that such a common and inexpensive drug can be used to increase and prolong the quality of life by treating such serious diseases is truly exciting."[46]

Hallmark 2: Decreased Glucose Levels in the Brain

Looking deeper into the dysfunctional metabolism seen in dementia, a study at the Lewis Katz School of Medicine at Temple

University in Philadelphia reports that one of the earliest signs of Alzheimer's disease is a decline in glucose levels in the brain.[47]

"In recent years, advances in imaging techniques, especially positron emission tomography (PET), have allowed researchers to look for subtle changes in the brains of patients with different degrees of cognitive impairment," explained Domenico Praticò, MD, Professor in the Center for Translational Medicine at the Lewis Katz School of Medicine at Temple University (LKSOM). "One of the changes that has been consistently reported is a decrease in glucose availability in the hippocampus."

Based on these findings, all forms of dementia and neurodegeneration could accurately be called diabetes of the brain, a situation in which brain cells cannot use glucose. So what role (if any) can methylene blue play in restoring glucose use by cells?

A 2015 study reports that treating astrocytes, the star-shaped glial cells in the brain and spinal cord that are essential for brain function, with methylene blue "significantly increased cellular oxygen consumption, glucose uptake, and ATP production."[48]

Methylene Blue and Red Light Therapy for Dementia

When it comes to therapies for diseases of the brain, two stand out among the crowd as the most promising. Methylene blue and red light therapy are two widely studied approaches for improving brain mitochondrial respiration due to their ability to act directly on cellular metabolism and correct deficiencies therein. Red light and methylene blue "have similar beneficial effects on mitochondrial function, oxidative damage, inflammation, and subsequent behavioral symptoms," a 2020 review reports.[49] Combining methylene blue with red light therapy in a treatment protocol for dementia appears to be a promising technique for synergistically maximizing therapeutic potency and accelerating recovery of metabolically defective brain cells.

5. Cognitive Enhancement: A Brain-Boosting Powerhouse

It wasn't until about 100 years after discovering methylene blue that scientists began realizing its immense potential to improve brain function. A 1970s animal study revealed improved memory in rats after ingesting the substance. Further explorations into the effects of methylene blue on the brain didn't occur until many decades later. Once they began, reports coming out were every bit as promising, even in humans.

In recent years, methylene blue has gained popularity among 'self-hackers' and nootropic enthusiasts as a brain-boosting compound used to enhance cognition. The tendency of this dye to quickly cross the blood-brain barrier and concentrate inside the brain makes it the perfect candidate for therapy to enhance brain function. Once inside, methylene blue improves mitochondrial efficiency and protects brain cells from damage through its antioxidant functions, resulting in improved memory, mood, and overall cognition.

A Single Oral Dose Improves Memory and Attention

Dr. Timothy Duong and his colleagues at the University of Texas Health Science Center conducted the very first human study investigating the impact of methylene blue on memory and attention span in 2016.[50] The randomized, double-blind, placebo-controlled clinical trial administered an oral dose (0.5-4.0mg/kg) of methylene blue to twenty-six healthy participants between the ages 22 and 62 to determine if the substance could increase brain activity and improve performance in memory- and attention-related tasks.

Participants underwent functional magnetic resonance imaging (MRI) before and one hour after low-dose methylene blue or placebo was administered to evaluate the effects of methylene blue on cerebrovascular activity during tasks. The study found that a single oral dose of methylene blue improved both short-term memory and attention span in the participants. "Methylene blue was also associated with a 7% increase in correct responses during memory retrieval," the study reports.

"This work certainly provides a foundation for future trials of methylene blue in healthy aging, cognitive impairment, dementia and other conditions that might benefit from drug-induced memory enhancement," Dr. Duong said.[51]

Methylene Blue Increases Mitochondrial Complex I-III Function

One of the hallmarks of dementia, as mentioned previously, is reduced mitochondrial complex IV, the activity of which can be enhanced by using methylene blue. But what about complexes I to III? This has been studied: "MB significantly increases mitochondrial complex I–III activity in isolated mitochondria and enhances oxygen consumption and glucose uptake."[52] Methylene blue targets all four complexes in the mitochondrial respiratory chain, which explains the brain-boosting benefits of this remarkable therapeutic blue dye.

NO Accelerates Cognitive Decline, MB Prevents it

One final mechanism for the cognitive benefits of methylene blue is that reducing nitric oxide in the brain has been found to be protective against cognitive decline. "Overall our findings suggest that lack of NO release via nNOS may protect animals to some extent against age-associated cognitive decline in memory tasks..."[53] Methylene blue, a nitric oxide inhibitor, maintains efficient cellular metabolism in brain cells, protecting the brain from dementia and age-related decline.

6. Depression No More

More than 264 million individuals worldwide currently suffer from clinical depression, but these are only the officially-diagnosed numbers. The truth is, we all suffer from bouts of depression at different points in our lives, and so wouldn't it be useful to understand what is happening inside the body during depression and how to take care of the problem?

Many people with depression are prescribed SSRI drugs. But, with an endless list of serious side effects such as weight gain, insomnia, sexual dysfunction, emotional detachment, drowsiness, anxiety, restlessness, agitation, tremors, headaches, blurred vision, mania, psychosis, hallucinations, suicide and homicidal ideation, isn't it safe for us to say that they don't work? Unbeknownst to the public, scientists have known for many years that the root cause of depression is *not* a deficiency of the neurotransmitter serotonin.

The Serotonin Hypothesis is *WRONG!*

The "serotonin hypothesis" of clinical depression has been around for more than 50 years and claims that serotonin deficiency is the cause of depression. This hypothesis is the backbone to the entire line of SSRI drug treatments used by millions of people worldwide. But there's a problem – the serotonin hypothesis has never been proven. In fact, the idea that inadequate serotonin causes depression is so far from reality that in a 2015 review, scientists called the serotonin hypothesis a conspiracy theory pushed by drug manufacturers to sell drugs to a gullible public.[54]

"Dogged by unreliable clinical biochemical findings and the difficulty of relating changes in serotonin activity to mood state, the serotonin hypothesis eventually achieved 'conspiracy theory' status, whose avowed purpose was to enable industry to market selective serotonin reuptake inhibitors (SSRIs) to a gullible public." The pharmaceutical industry is duping anybody taking SSRI drugs, and their health and quality of life likely decreased, solely for financial gain.

Hopefully, the new paradigm on depression and its solutions that I'm about to offer have an anti-depressant effect on you after that last point.

Serotonin: Molecule of Aggression, Depression, and Stress

Would it surprise you if I told you 'the happy hormone' serotonin is not a hormone at all? Or that serotonin is involved in *causing* depression? How about if I said that people with Cancer had elevated serotonin?

The failed 'serotonin hypothesis' suggests that serotonin is *not* involved in making people feel 'happy,' and its long list of serious side effects tells us that it's working in ways not conducive to health. So long as billions of dollars are being made selling SSRI drugs, the evening news, unfortunately, will never broadcast the case against them. This makes you wonder how long it will take before the world realizes serotonin is, in fact, what Ray Peat calls "a damage-induced inflammatory mediator" involved in aggression, depression, and stress.

"Reserpine is an ancient tranquilizer, derived from a plant used in India for centuries. It has a powerful tranquilizing action, has been used to treat hypertension, and was found to be an antidepressant (Davies and Shepherd, 1955). It lowers the concentration of serotonin in the brain and other tissues."
- Dr. Raymond Peat.

The Role of Stress in Depression

For many decades, stress has been known to trigger symptoms of depression. In January 2021, United States and Chinese researchers collaborated on a study published in the journal *Translational Psychiatry,* which investigated adolescent depression using a non-human primate stress-induced model of depression. The monkeys faced stressors such as water deprivation, fasting, space restrictions, cold stress, strobe light, and inescapable footshocks. The study confirmed that chronic and unpredictable mild stressors could induce depressive-like and anxiety-like behavior while increasing the stress hormone cortisol and reducing metabolic rate.[55]

Three primary biological consequences of stress in the study include:

1. Stress *caused* depression and anxiety
2. Stress *increased* stress hormone cortisol
3. Stress *reduced* metabolic rate

There's no doubt that our modern lives are riddled with mild chronic stressors, and at times, severe chronic stressors - and these stressors are contributing to the epidemic of depression in ourselves and the people around us. The study I presented above brings us full circle to what can be declared the primary cause of depression.

Depression is a Metabolic Disease

The brain is unique in that it is strictly dependent on glucose to meet its metabolic energy needs. It's also unique because, relative to other parts of the body, the brain requires proportionally far more energy for its weight than the rest of the body. While the brain typically makes up around 2% of a person's weight, it consumes around 20% of the body's energy – and that's when at rest! While reading, exercising, or performing any cognitively-demanding activity, brain cells consume far more energy. In fact, the brain consumes 10 times the rate of energy per gram of tissue than the rest of the body.

When glucose, being the major fuel for brain cell metabolism, is in short supply, the energy supply to the brain is quickly cut off. It's in this metabolically-depressed state that a person begins experiencing all the feelings, the behaviors, and the signs and symptoms of *depression*.

A 2017 study published in *PLoS One* shows an association between poor metabolic health and depression.[56] In a large, diverse cohort of adults studied in 2018, the presence of depression was associated with dysfunctional metabolic health.[57] Scientific explorations into depression have taken us a long way, disproving the false serotonin hypothesis, and bringing us to what is becoming increasingly more established and obvious as time goes on: depression is a metabolic disorder.

"We see an unexpected link between cellular energetics and major depression, which has always been seen as a mood disorder," states Professor Fliny, a professor of molecular psychiatry at the University of Oxford, UK.[58]

Why Depression is More Common in Women than in Men

Harvard Medical School reports that "women are about twice as likely as men to develop major depression."[59] This finding was based on a large-scale 2017 study that found these gender differences in depression begin at age 12, with girls and women being twice as likely as men to experience depression.[60]

But even the prestigious Harvard University doesn't offer much in the way of reasons why women are more prone to depression, stating, "It remains unclear why a gender gap exists in depression." Step aside, Harvard, and let the independent health researcher offer some clarity on the issue.

The reason why depression is more common in women than in men is the same reason why migraine headaches are 2-3 times more prevalent in women, or why autoimmune diseases are as much as 10 times more prevalent in women: women have higher levels of estrogen. It's no coincidence that as estrogen levels peak during a woman's menstrual cycle around days 22-24, the prevalence of depression has been found also to proportionally increase.

Here are four specific biological pathways that help explain why depression is more common in women in men (four ways estrogen causes depression):

1. **Estrogen Increases Serotonin** – One consequence of estrogen exposure is that it increases the production of serotonin. "These results suggest that estrogen may increase the capacity for serotonin synthesis," concluded researchers from the University of Washington.[61]

2. **Estrogen Increases Cortisol** – In a 2007 study investigating the impact of taking oral estrogen on 37 women, serum concentrations of the stress hormone cortisol were found to be 67% higher than in control subjects.[62] Cortisol is a hormone of stress, and stress causes depression.

3. **Estrogen Suppresses Thyroid** – Estrogen causes increased levels of polyunsaturated free fatty acids to circulate in the bloodstream. Polyunsaturated fatty acids suppress the immune system, inhibit cellular respiration, and powerfully suppress thyroid function. The end results of estrogen-induced hypothyroidism are the inability of cells to oxidize glucose and *a lower metabolic rate*, which have been linked directly to depression.

4. **Estrogen Increases Nitric Oxide** – Estrogen is well-known to induce nitric oxide production via the activation of the enzyme nitric oxide synthase,[63] and it turns out nitric oxide plays a critical role in depression.

Nitric Oxide is Central to Depression

To truly understand depression, it's necessary to step back from the cultural beliefs surrounding serotonin and neurotransmitters and look at the larger biological picture.

While the public, medical doctors, some scientists, and even naturopaths are taught to see nitric oxide (NO) through a one-dimensional lens – as a factor for greater blood flow in the brain and body – they fail to realize that "Low concentrations of NO are neuroprotective and mediate physiological signaling whereas higher concentrations mediate neuroinflammatory actions and are neurotoxic."[64]

When nitric oxide is increased in the brain and body, increased also are two different free radicals – reactive nitrogen species and reactive oxygen species. This results in greater production of pro-inflammatory cytokines. Nitric oxide is responsible for initiating the high levels of inflammation commonly found in depressed people. Brain on fire!

Based on these findings, we should expect depressed people to have higher nitric oxide levels than non-depressed people. This research has been done: In rats and humans with major depressive disorder, "plasma NO levels were significantly increased both in male CUS rats and in male MDD patients."[65] In another study, the severity of psychomotor retardation seen in people with major depression was significantly correlated to the serum nitric oxide level.[66]

Nitric Oxide Inhibitors as Anti-Depressants

In recent years, nitric oxide *inhibitors* have been studied as anti-depressants. Targeting nitric oxide appears to be a far more promising target for treating depression than serotonin or other neurotransmitters, since nitric oxide regulates neurotransmitter expression and the release of pro-inflammatory cytokines.

In rats, inhibiting nitric oxide has anti-depressant like effects in the forced swimming test, which means it helped them maintain hope and continue to swim, instead of giving up and drowning. If you think of life as a kind of "forced swimming test," it means these results could be very applicable to our modern lives.[67]

All things prior in this section have led us to methylene blue – the star of the show – a drug known for its ability to potently inhibit nitric oxide production in numerous ways, which has been used in psychiatry for over a century.

Methylene Blue: A Cure for Depression?

Scientists gave severely depressed patients one dose of methylene blue daily for three weeks and "Improvement in patients receiving methylene blue was significantly greater than in those receiving a placebo." Remarkably, the significant improvements were achieved in the patients at the minute dose of only 15 mg/day.[68]

Methylene Blue for Bipolar Disorder

Formerly called manic depression, bipolar disorder is a mental health condition that causes extreme mood swings that include emotional highs and lows. Methylene blue has been put to the test on patients with bipolar disorder, beginning in the 1980s. More trials have occurred in recent years as interest in this valuable medicine is rekindled.

A 2-year trial on 31 bipolar patients compared 300mg/day of methylene blue with 15mg/day methylene blue in 1986. All patients were also treated using lithium. Of the 17 patients that completed the 2-year trial, they were significantly less depressed when on 300mg/day methylene blue compared to 15mg/day. The 300mg/day dose was said to be "a useful addition to lithium in the long-term treatment of manic-depressive psychosis."[69]

It's important to note that taking lithium, the standard treatment for bipolar at that time, can come with serious potential consequences, like tremors, acne, nausea, excessive salivation, weight gain, memory defects, kidney failure, a 6-fold increased risk of hypothyroidism, and abnormally large production of urine (polyuria). I think it's safe to say the improvements in patients in the study mentioned above would probably have been more significant if they hadn't also been taking lithium.

Dalhousie University in Halifax, Canada, was the launchpad of a 2017 study that tested the bipolar drug lamotrigine, used in conjunction with methylene blue. Patients took lamotrigine with methylene blue at a dose of either 15mg or 195mg for three months, then switched to the other dose of methylene blue for three more months. Treatment involving 195mg of methylene blue "improved residual symptoms of depression and anxiety in patients with bipolar disorder," concluded the researchers.[70] Several of the patients in the study liked methylene blue so much that they continued using it after the study was complete.

Methylene Blue Eliminates Negative Feelings About The Past

One of the most unique and fascinating brain benefits of methylene blue is its ability to release negative feelings associated with past situations, allowing the user to retain the positive aspects of those events and 'move on' from fears or trauma. In the scientific world, they call this 'fear extincttion.' In the real world, the people who need these kinds of therapies have Post-Traumatic Stress Disorder (PTSD). I realize this topic drifts slightly from the subject of depression. Still, there's definitely some overlap between depression and how people with PTSD experience the world, which is why I've decided to include it.

In 2014, scientists administered methylene blue to people with a marked fear of claustrophobia to determine if it could help extinguish their fears. For the study, published in the *American Journal of Psychiatry*, subjects were crammed inside tiny, dark chambers six times for five minutes each time, followed immediately by administration of either methylene blue (260mg) or a placebo. They repeated the process one month later and assessed the level of fear in the participants.

The study found that participants who had "successful exposure sessions" (fairly low levels of fear after spending time in enclosed chambers) had even lower levels of fear the second time around if they received methylene blue. Interestingly, patients who had "unsuccessful exposure sessions," (high levels of fear after spending time in enclosed chambers) fared worse on follow-up after receiving methylene blue. The results of this study were a little less satisfying than I had hoped, but still in some ways promising. "Methylene blue enhances memory and the retention of fear extinction when administered after a successful exposure session but may have a deleterious effect on extinction when administered after an unsuccessful exposure session," concluded researchers.[71]

More recent studies using methylene blue for fear extinction have reported positive effects in preventing fear reinstatement in certain subgroups of animals.[72] A 2017 randomized controlled trial on humans with chronic Post Traumatic Stress Disorder found that methylene blue, in addition to imaginary exposure therapy (imagining yourself holding that King Cobra snake you fear), successfully accelerated fear extinction recovery in patients with chronic PTSD.[73]

This section was so vast that I created a summary of all the information included before we move on. Below are the findings from the most recent review of methylene blue for brain disorders in an easy-to-digest point-form fashion. A 2019 review[74] of methylene blue for neuropsychiatric disorders reports:

- Methylene blue has antidepressant, anxiolytic, and neuroprotective properties.

- Methylene blue has a stabilizing effect on mitochondrial function.

- "Particularly promising results have been obtained in both short- and long-term treatment of bipolar disorder."

- Methylene blue is effective for psychotic and mood disorders and can help with fear extinction.

7. Hope for Autism

The other day my sister sent me a text saying her friend's daughter was "on the Autism spectrum," which inspired me to investigate Autism and include a section about it in this book. My goal was to learn what Autism is and determine if methylene blue therapy can help people with Autism.

Autism Prevalence Rising Exponentially

Autism is the fastest-growing developmental disability in the United States. If that's not concerning enough, then here are a couple more alarming facts: 1) Autism is mostly diagnosed in children, and 2) its prevalence has been increasing exponentially for the past 50 years. The following chart illustrates the statistics on Autism prevalence between the years 1975 and 2009.

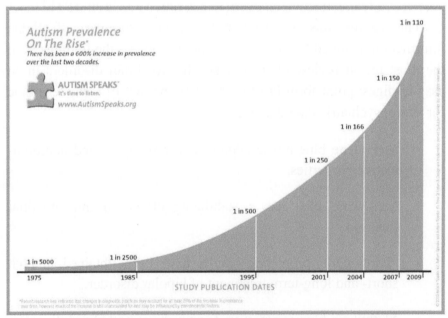

Autism prevalence between 1975 and 2009. Autismspeaks.org

As you can see, in 1975, 1 in 5000 children was diagnosed with Autism, which is not many at all; it was a rare disorder then. But just ten years later, that figure doubled to 1 in 2500, and by 1995, the number skyrocketed to 1 in 500. In 2001, Autism prevalence was 1 in 250 children, and in 2009 – the last year of data available at the time the above graph was created – prevalence of Autism was 1 in 110 children. I wish I could say that's where the numbers stopped climbing, but statistics show that the cases have continued their exponential climb since then.

Autism prevalence released by the CDC for the year 2020 pegs rates among children at *1 in 54 children* in the United States. To put it into perspective, we've gone from 1 in 5000 children with Autism in 1975 to 1 in 54 children in 2020. Why isn't anybody solving this disease? F*ck it, I'll do it. Let's go!

Symptoms of Autism

We're all born with greatness inside of us, but because of the crippling social effects seen in people with this Autism, children or adults with the disease fail to forge the relationships and cognitive capacity needed to live in a way that is fulfilling to themselves and has a positive impact on others around them.

Symptoms of Autism include…

- Avoidance of eye contact

- Not working or playing well with others

- Absence of facial expressions

- Avoidance of physical contact

- Confusion regarding their own emotions and the emotions of others

- General distress while being around other people

There's no way we can have a healthy, functioning society with a large percentage of the population walking around with these kinds of social issues. People with Autism generally are unable to take care of themselves, which means when a child has Autism, their parents and all caregivers for the remainder of their lives must spend virtually every waking moment taking care of them. The impact of this on individual lives, families, and society is probably more significant than we can imagine – and it means that when one individual suffers from Autism, we all suffer. Understanding the true nature of the disease and how to eliminate it would be a priceless gift for countless lives and humankind.

I'm here to bring you a message of hope for Autism: there's a good chance methylene blue will one day be crowned the ultimate therapy for Autism Spectrum Disorder in people of all ages, genders, and races.

Autism: A Metabolic Disorder?

According to the World Health Organization, "There are probably many factors that make a child more likely to have ASD [Autism Spectrum Disorder], including environmental and genetic factors." Well, fair enough, but it's 2021. If astronauts could land on the moon over 50 years ago, why the h*ll can't the medical industry come up with a therapeutic intervention to heal Autism? Instead, mainstream sources tell us, "There is no cure for Autism spectrum disorder, and there's currently no medication to treat it."[75]

By now, we know that methylene blue – rapidly and in many different ways – helps correct dysfunctional metabolism within all cells and tissues of the body. The question that needs to be asked is whether there's a relationship between ASD and metabolic dysfunction?

Looking at the existing scientific literature to find out, I discovered that evidence has been mounting for decades suggesting that Autism Spectrum Disorder is a metabolic disease.

In 2010, scientists at the University of California, Davis, published a landmark study that found children with Autism are *far more likely* to have deficits in their ability to produce cellular energy than healthy children.[76] "The various dysfunctions we measured are probably even more extreme in brain cells, which rely exclusively on mitochondria for energy," said Isaac Pessah, director of the Center for Children's Environmental Health and Disease Prevention, a UC Davis MIND Institute researcher, and professor of molecular biosciences at the UC Davis School of Veterinary Medicine.

One thing known to occur when cellular mitochondrial metabolism fails within cells is free radical electrons begin leaking from the respiratory chain, causing damage to intracellular components and organelles, including the mitochondria themselves. This explains why Giulivi and her colleagues found that hydrogen peroxide levels in autistic children were twice as high as children who did not have Autism. As a result, the cells of those with Autism were exposed to higher oxidative stress, which is one of the hallmarks of the disease.

"The real challenge now is to try and understand the role of mitochondrial dysfunction in children with Autism," Pessah said. "For instance, many environmental stressors can cause mitochondrial damage."[77]

The Role of Lipopolysaccharide in Autism

One phenomenon that has been powerfully linked to Autistic children is gut disorders. In 2020, a study by scientists at Duke University, Eastern Virginia Medical School, and Ohio State University found that increased severity of Autism symptoms was associated with more severe constipation, stomach pain, and other gut difficulties.[78] "In Autism, we wonder if the gut problems children experience are a core part of the disease itself or whether they're brought on by other symptoms that children with Autism experience," said the study's lead author Payal Chakraborty.[79] These scientists don't appear to understand the link between gut issues and Autism, so I'll offer a very important theory that I first encountered while reading the work of Dr. Raymond Peat.

Endotoxin, chemically known as lipopolysaccharide, is a poison produced by gram negative bacteria in the gut. I maintain that excess production of endotoxin in Autistic children is one of the most foundational reasons for the metabolic dysfunction seen in Autism.

My goal here is to keep things brief, so below, I'm presenting some important evidence in support of the endotoxin theory of Autism to give you a window into some of the research:

- Endotoxin injections induce inflammation and lesions in the white matter of the fetal brain.[80]

- Endotoxin promotes nitric oxide production and causes neuro-inflammation and cognitive impairment.[81]

- Endotoxin induces a depressive syndrome, characterized by the inability to feel pleasure (anhedonia), anorexia, and reduced locomotor, exploratory, and social behavior. This syndrome has been so well established that scientists have coined the term "Endotoxemia" to describe it.[82] [83] [84]

- Mercury and other heavy metals synergize with endotoxin and increase damage.[85]

- Endotoxin decreases glutathione levels, making it more difficult for the body to detoxify heavy metals.[86]

On the main page of their website, Microbialinfluence.com lists the many shocking similarities between Autism Spectrum Disorder and Lipopolysaccharide poisoning related to the brain, emotions and behavior, digestive issues, immune function, and more. Autism and endotoxin poisoning are virtually identical! This means that potentially dramatic improvements in children with Autism may result after the removal of endotoxin from their guts.

How to Reduce Endotoxin

To reduce endotoxin production in the gut, you must first understand how endotoxin is formed. Here's how it works…

Anytime food that your body cannot digest is consumed, that food sits in the gut and provides food for bacteria. After bacteria consume it, endotoxin is produced and excreted as a byproduct of bacterial metabolism. That endotoxin then wreaks havoc on the gut lining, causing all the gut problems that Autistic children experience as a core of the disease. The endotoxin then makes its way into the bloodstream and into tissues of the brain and body, negatively affecting every cell with which it interacts. The ideal amount of endotoxin in the body is zero; the less, the better. So how can we stop or slow its production?

There are two ways to reduce endotoxin production in the gut:

1. Reduce or eliminate consumption of the foods that promote endotoxin production.
2. Ingest antibiotic foods, drugs, or other substances to kill the bacteria so they cannot convert fiber and starch into endotoxin.

1. Eliminate endotoxin-producing foods

Foods that are good food for bacteria are all the ones that the human gut can't digest. Fiber/cellulose and starches are the primary culprits and can be found in raw plants, beans, grains, potatoes, and other starches.

After years of experimentation, I definitely think these foods can be a part of a healthy diet. But in a child with Autism, it's probably wise to remove them from the diet entirely during recovery.

For those who enjoy eating raw salads, I thought I would mention that cooking vegetables well before eating them is a great way to break down the undigestible cellulose inside them, which reduces endotoxin production and also makes them more digestible and nutritious.

2. Endotoxin Defeating Foods and Drugs

The second way to prevent endotoxin production is to take anti-bacterial drugs or other substances that eliminate the bacteria from the gut. By using this strategy, anytime you consume fibrous foods, you are wiping out the bacteria that would normally convert fiber into endotoxin.

The antibiotic minocycline, for example, has been shown to protect against lipopolysaccharide-induced cognitive impairment.[87]

Carrots are another example. Carrots produce their own mild anti-biotics to combat the bacteria and other microorganisms living in the soil in which they grow. In an article on Endalldisease.com called *A Raw Carrot A Day Keeps the Doctor Away*, I discuss some scientific research showing the benefits of raw carrot on the gut.

"One vegetable has a special place in a diet to balance the hormones, and that is the raw carrot. It is so nearly indigestible that, when it is well chewed or grated, it helps to stimulate the intestine and reduce the reabsorption of estrogen and the absorption of bacterial toxins. In these effects on the bowel, which improve hormonal balance, a carrot salad resembles antibiotic therapy, except that the carrot salad can be used every day for years without harmful side-effects. Many people find that daily use of the raw carrot eliminates their PMS, headaches, or allergies.

The use of oil and vinegar as dressing intensifies the bowel-cleansing effect of the salad. Coconut oil is more germicidal and thyroid promoting than olive oil, but a mixture of coconut and olive oil improves the flavor. Lime juice. salt, cheese and meats can be used to vary the flavor." - **Dr. Raymond Peat**

Methylene blue, although antibacterial, will be absorbed long before it has the chance to kill endotoxin-producing gut bacteria in the colon, but it can exert rapid neuroprotective effects on lipopolysaccharide-induced behavioral deficits.[88] Red light therapy is also protective against the damage induced by lipopolysaccharide.[89]

Activated charcoal is another inexpensive medicinal that can be used to wipe out gut bacteria in children with Autism. It is highly antibacterial, and its oral consumption has shown to result in a significant reduction in lipopolysaccharide levels in the blood.[90]

Contrary to the 'gut microbiome' theory and the companies trying to sell us $20 bottles of probiotics, the ideal situation in the gut appears to be complete sterilization. This explains why rats that lived their entire lives with sterile guts, maintained through feeding of activated charcoal at every meal, were found to live 43% longer than rats with bacterially populated guts.[91] It also explains why tetracycline and other antibiotics have been found to have powerful anti-tumor properties. Reduced endotoxin production is the mechanism in both cases, which benefits the body by reducing the body's exposure to metabolic inhibiting endotoxin.

Autism: The Metabolic Disease Unravelled

Let's take a stroll down memory lane and I'll show you some of the scientific evidence published within the past decade or so linking Autism Spectrum Disorder [ASD] directly to mitochondrial dysfunction.

- **2012:** "One of the medical disorders that has been consistently associated with ASD [Autism Spectrum Disorder] is mitochondrial dysfunction."[92]

- **2013:** "We show two clinical cases of ASD associated to a deficiency of the mitochondrial respiratory chain (complex I+III and IV)."[93]

- **2014:** Lactate significantly higher in brains of children with Autism.[94]

- **2015:** Large numbers of children with Autism demonstrate abnormalities in mitochondrial function as well as gastrointestinal symptoms, and interestingly, GI symptoms are also common in children with mitochondrial disorders.[95]

- **2016 Review:** "Overall, the findings support the hypothesis that there is an association of ASD [Autism Spectrum Disorder] with impaired mitochondrial function."[96]

Not only is the link between Autism and mitochondrial dysfunction overwhelmingly evident at this point, but one of the most recent findings was that the number of Autistic children with disrupted energy metabolism is actually *much* higher than previously thought. While it was once believed that around 5% of children with Autism had mitochondrial dysfunction, recent research from Columbia University has revealed the actual percentage is as high as 80%!

Karen K Griffiths and Richard J. Levy, from the Department of Anesthesiology at Columbia University Medical Center in New York, New York, USA, reported in 2020 that "abnormalities of mitochondrial function could affect a much higher number of children with ASD, perhaps up to 80%."[97] I think researchers will eventually realize that metabolic issues are universal in Autism Spectrum Disorder.

Targeting Cellular Mitochondria in Autism

The Electron Transport Chain is series of four protein complexes that exist within the membrane of the mitochondria and are responsible for Oxidative Phosphorylation (OxPhos)—the main method through which ATP is produced.

Deficits in the mitochondrial transport chain exist almost universally in Autism. For example, in the two clinical cases mentioned above, a deficiency in complexes I, III, and IV were found. Remarkably, methylene blue can act as an alternative electron carrier and bypass these defects at any and all of the four complexes.

"MB significantly increases mitochondrial complex I–III activity"[98], and "MB increases mitochondrial complex IV by 30%."[99]

"As I have shown in my earlier days, one can knock out the whole respiratory chain by cyanide and then restore oxygen uptake by adding methylene blue which takes the whole electron transport over between dehydrogenases and O_2." **–Albert Szent-Györgi**

By using methylene blue to restore the mitochondrial complexes, lactate production (glycolysis) is switched *off* and replaced by the full oxidative phosphorylation of glucose into ATP, and the body's primary vasodilator and antioxidant, carbon dioxide. Carbon dioxide intensifies oxygen uptake and use by cells via The Bohr Effect, further enhancing the body's metabolic rate. And in the pursuit of health and healing, a high metabolic rate means we've reached the summit.

8. The Great Pain Reliever

Pain experiments using methylene blue on prison inmates date back to 1890. An article published by Dr. Paul Ehrlich and Arthur Leppmann in the German medical journal *Deutsche Medizinische Wochenschrift*, describes administering a young, mentally ill male prison inmate methylene blue for pain.[100] Remarkably, the researchers found that methylene blue changed the entire state of the nerves. Just a few hours after subcutaneous injection or oral administration of methylene blue, painful inflammation of nerves subsided extraordinarily, often entirely with further injections.

Since that study, much research has been done on methylene blue's ability to relieve pain in different afflictions, such as postoperative pain caused by surgery, chronic shooting pain, oral mucositis caused by chemotherapy, arthritis, migraine headaches, and chronic low back pain. We will explore all of these now.

Methylene Blue for Surgical Pain

Surgery to remove haemorrhoids is called haemorrhoidectomy and has been associated with considerable postoperative pain and discomfort. In a 2014 trial, doctors tested the impact of injecting methylene blue under the skin surrounding the anus before slicing off haemorrhoids. Group 1 received injections with the anesthetic marcaine and saline before surgical dissection, and Group 2 received injections of marcaine and methylene blue. "The mean pain scores were significantly lower and the use of paracetamol [acetaminophen] was also significantly less in the methylene blue group during the first three postoperative days," the study reports, and concluded that methylene blue "was useful in reducing the initial postoperative pain of open haemorrhoidectomy."[101]

Methylene Blue for Chronic Neuropathic Pain

Chronic neuropathic pain is often described as a shooting or burning pain, caused by dysfunction in the nervous system as the result of trauma, infection, or a restriction in blood supply to tissues (ischemia). Sometimes it is relentless and severe, and sometimes it comes and goes.

In 2015, Scientists from the Multidisciplinary Pain Clinic at Uppsala University Hospital in Sweden conducted a clinical trial testing methylene blue on patients with neuropathic pain. Ten patients were randomized to either receive methylene blue or placebo. Results show that within 60 minutes of administration, patients who received methylene blue experienced pain relief, and over the next 48 hours after administration, the decrease in pain was significant.[102]

Methylene Blue for Oral Mucositis

Oral mucositis is a common and debilitating side effect of chemo-therapy and radiotherapy treatments for Cancer that manifests in the form of painful inflammation and ulceration of the mucous membranes in the mouth.

In 2021, Carlos J Roldan and his colleagues at the University of Texas gave an oral methylene blue mouth rinse to 281 Cancer patients with oral mucositis. Pain scores were reduced from 7.7 to 2.5 after methylene blue oral rinse, and most patients achieved pain control after the first three doses. This led the researchers to conclude, "MB oral rinse is an effective and safe treatment for refractory pain from oral mucositis related to Cancer treatment."[103]

Methylene Blue for Arthritis Pain

Anyone suffering from arthritis knows how debilitating it is to have slow-moving and painful joints and how much it can affect your overall quality of life. Thankfully, research using methylene blue to treat arthritis is highly promising.

In a 2018 study at Wuhan University in China, Li, Tang, Wang, and their team of scientists injected methylene blue into the knee joints of rabbits and analyzed the results. Remarkably, the treatment "significantly enhanced the weight distribution and significantly decreased the swelling ratio of the rabbits." The study concluded that methylene blue was effective for relieving arthritis-associated pain and inflammation.[104]

Arthritis progression often results in degraded cartilage in the joints, causing increased pain, immobility, and inflammation. It turns out, arthritic cartilage discs excrete 10x as much nitric oxide as non-arthritic cartilage discs, and this excess nitric oxide mediates cartilage degradation.

In a 2000 study, Israeli scientists wrote "Nitric oxide (NO) appears to be a final common inflammation mediator of cartilage degradation." The great nitric oxide-inhibiting drug methylene blue was tested to see if it could have a preservation effect on the cartilage matrix. The study shows that the "Addition of methylene blue to the growth medium lowered nitric oxide accumulation and prevented matrix degradation in the cultured cartilage discs."[105]

Methylene Blue for Migraine Headaches

Increased nitric oxide has been heavily implicated in migraine headaches in recent research. A 2018 review on the subject highlights the role of nitric oxide in headaches and recommends using nitric oxide synthase inhibitors to treat this disorder.[106] Methylene blue's ability to potently inhibit nitric oxide production and scavenge existing nitric oxide from the body and blood make it a drug of great interest and promise for those in search of evidence-based treatment for migraine headaches.

Methylene Blue for Low Back Pain

One of the most remarkable studies ever conducted on low back pain came from the General Hospital of Armed Police Force in Beijing in 2010. The study showed strong evidence that the injection of methylene blue into a painful disc is a "safe, effective, and minimally invasive" method for the treatment of discogenic low back pain, far more effective than any other known treatment for low back pain.[107] Of the 72 patients enrolled in the study, 36 were given a placebo and 36 were given methylene blue injections directly into the spinal discs experiencing pain. The results showed that of the 36 patients given methylene blue injections, 19% were completely pain free, and 72% almost completely pain free. Said differently, over 90% of patients experienced total or near-total relief!

Low back pain expert Nikolai Bogkduk wrote in an editorial that he sees "no lethal flaws in the study" and calls it "one of the most incredible studies on low back pain treatment ever published." The results he described as "astounding, unprecedented and unrivalled in the history of research into the treatment of chronic discogenic low back pain." Methylene blue could make spinal surgery "essentially obsolete" and would be "worthy of nomination for a Nobel Prize," proclaimed Bogkduk.[108]

In the study, satisfaction rates of the methylene blue treatment group were 91.6% compared to a dismal 0.70%, 1.68%, and 14.3%, respectively, in the placebo treatment group. There were no side effects or complications in patients treated with methylene blue.

"Intradiskal injection of methylene blue can substantially decrease pain scores and improve function for discogenic back pain," was the conclusion of a 2021 meta-analysis on the use of methylene blue for low back pain.

The pain-relieving effects of methylene blue are rapid and profound. As we've seen in this section, the remarkable drug methylene blue appears helpful for many, if not all, types of physical pain.

9. A Healthier Heart

Fundamental to your health and life is the quality of your beating heart and cardiovascular system, which circulate nourishing blood through your vessels to all parts of the body and back again. Some interesting scientific findings have been uncovered in recent years regarding the interactions of nitric oxide, blood vessel quality, and aging of the heart.

In elderly patients with hypertension, significantly elevated levels of nitric oxide have been found,[109] which suggests that nitric oxide may affect longevity. In animal studies, scientists have seen it firsthand: Overexpression of the major enzyme that manufactures nitric oxide, nitric oxide synthase (iNOS), significantly increases mortality.[110] This increased mortality was associated with enlarged heart and excessive dilation of heart ventricles, as well as a high incidence of sudden death caused by bradyarrythmia – a very slow heart rate below 60bpm. These are some of the harmful things that excessive nitric oxide can do to your cardiovascular system, and what nitric oxide inhibiting substances like methylene blue can help remedy.

For example, give an old rat a nitric oxide inhibitor, and it can promote relaxed more youthful blood vessels.[111] "Aging-associated vascular oxidative stress is partially reversed by pharmacological NOS inhibition," wrote Johns Hopkins Hospital researchers in 2009.

This finding was reinforced in human subjects in 2011 when Caroline J Smith and her fellow scientists from the Department of Kinesiology at Pennsylvania State University discovered increased iNOS expression in blood vessels of hypertensive patients. Administering an iNOS inhibitor restored vasodilation in hypertensive human patients.[112]

Oh No! Peroxynitrite (ONOO)

What is it about nitric oxide that causes the stiff vessels, enlarged heart, and cardiovascular dysfunction seen in animals and humans? One of the mechanisms talked about in the research is the increased production of a potent toxic chemical derived from the reaction between nitric oxide and oxygen, called peroxynitrite (ONOO).[113]

ONOO is a toxic free radical that's harmful to cellular lipids, genetic material, and proteins.[114] Scavenging the ONOO using antioxidants can restore endothelium-dependent dilation of arteries.

And therefore, contrary to what the many proponents of nitric oxide believe, the scientific evidence teaches us that increased nitric oxide constricts blood vessels and *lowering* NO (by inhibiting iNOS) can actually *restore* vasodilation in aged blood vessels.[115]

The Role of Endotoxin in Heart Disease

In the section of this chapter on Autism, you learned about the bacterially-derived poison called endotoxin. It's important to mention that this ubiquitous poison is one of the leading contributors, not just to the pathology of Autism but to virtually all metabolic diseases, including cardiovascular disease.

In a study from 2000, when scientists injected lipopolysaccharide into rats, they witnessed levels of iNOS *soar!* Next, they injected methylene blue into the rats to see if it would be protective. The results speak for themselves: The induction of iNOS was "completely eliminated" in the presence of methylene blue.[116]

Endotoxin (lipopolysaccharide) is one potent way to activate the cytokine storm iNOS production in the cardiovascular system, which leads to coronary heart disease, report scientists McCann, Mastronardi, de Laurentiis, and Rettori in their 2005 review titled "The Nitric Oxide Theory of Aging Revisited."[117]

MB supplementation is highly protective of cardiovascular function in disease and aging. Through its action as a nitric-oxide inhibitor and antioxidant, methylene blue can prevent both the formation of new peroxynitrite and scavenge existing peroxynitrite, which has been implicated in the diseased and aged heart.

Heart damage is common in patients with diabetes. And if methylene blue is, in fact, protective to the heart, we should expect improved cardiac function in diabetic patients given methylene blue. When doctors administered methylene blue to a 66-year old diabetic woman after suffering a heart attack, she "made a full and rapid recovery following the introduction of a methylene blue infusion."[118]

Romanian scientists showed us in 2017 that methylene blue improves heart health by enhancing mitochondrial respiration and decreasing oxidative stress.[119] And since we've touched on the subject of diabetes: methylene blue has shown to prevent diabetes,[120] restore eye health in patients with diabetes,[121] and lower blood sugar in diabetes animal studies.[122] In other words, both cardiovascular disease and diabetes are metabolic disorders, and their root cause can be influenced positively by methylene blue.

10. Methylene Blue vs. Cancer

The metabolism of Cancer cells varies significantly from normal cells. Normal cells oxidize glucose within their mitochondria, and Cancer cells rely on the fermentation of sugar (aerobic glycolysis). However, once sugar is depleted from the bloodstream and sugar stores (glycogen) are depleted from the liver, Cancer cells begin consuming fatty acids and protein.[123] Cancer is a metabolic disease characterized by the inability of cells to oxidize glucose inside their mitochondria. The switch from normal cell metabolism to Cancer cell metabolism is called The Warburg Effect, which was first documented over 90 years ago by 2x Nobel Prize Winning German scientist Otto Heinrich Warburg.

What Cancer Isn't

The idea that when somebody is diagnosed with cancer we must kill the cancer before the cancer kills them, is a deadly and unscientific mythology that has resulted in the unnecessary suffering and death of millions of people. Only if a cancer cell or tumor is viewed as some kind of monster-like creature that's hell-belt on killing the patient can the use of knives, poison injections and ionizing radiation be justified as treatments. Yet, the mythology of what I like to call *The Angry Cancer Cell* is so pervasive in society that most medical doctors, scientists, and the general public believe it as if it were fact. This is probably why Dr. Dean Burke, who worked directly with Dr. Warburg for many years, said of the American Cancer Society, "They lie like scoundrels." Or why the co-discoverer of DNA, Dr. James Watson, said "The American public is being sold a nasty bill of goods about Cancer."

For over 100 years, it has been known that Cancer is not a genetic disease, but rather a disease of damaged metabolism within cells. With the proper interventions, Cancer cells can revert back to normal cells, *no killing necessary!*

The New Metabolic Cancer Treatment Paradigm

For decades, scientists have been churning out evidence showing that Cancer cell metabolism can be restored to normal cell metabolism. The only reason the public isn't aware of this information is that the predominant Cancer treatments of today – surgery, chemotherapy, and radiotherapy – generate far too much profit for the industry to admit the truth. If the Cancer industry admitted this information publicly, it would put itself out of business, forfeiting $126 Billion in annual revenue. All that's left to leave the disease of Cancer behind us forever is for the public is to read and understand the information written in the book *Cancer: The Metabolic Disease Unravelled.*

The book references over 30 studies showing Cancer cells transform back into normal cells. In one study, scientists put mitochondria from Cancer cells into normal cells and observed the normal cells transform into Cancer cells. When they put mitochondria from normal cells into Cancer cells, the Cancer cells transformed back into normal cells.[124]

In 1995, researchers from Ohio State University stated, "...our data suggest quite strongly that nonmalignant tumor populations can be converted to a more malignant phenotype without additional mutations taking place and, conversely, malignant populations can be downregulated to a nontumorigenic phenotype."[125]

Before looking at methylene blue as a treatment for Cancer, I'd like to outline the critical role that nitric oxide plays its formation, progression, and metastasis. Once the havoc wrought by nitric oxide is understood, methylene blue's value for Cancer and other diseases becomes clear.

Nitric Oxide is Central to Cancer

One way to turn a healthy cell into a Cancer cell is to expose it to the environmental pollutant nitric oxide. My book *The Cancer Industry* explains how nitric oxide can induce carcinogenesis, tumor growth, and Cancer metastasis. Below I've elucidated three ways nitric oxide can trigger carcinogenesis.

Nitric Oxide Inhibits Cytochrome c Oxidase (Complex IV)

The enzyme cytochrome c oxidase plays a critical role in healthy mitochondrial metabolism; it interacts directly with oxygen and catalyzes the final step in oxidative phosphorylation. Expose this essential respiratory enzyme to nitric oxide, and it becomes inhibited. By binding directly to cytochrome c oxidase, nitric oxide "flips" the metabolic "switch" from mitochondrial respiration to aerobic glycolysis, aka "Cancer." Only two known interventions are capable of dissociating nitric oxide from cytochrome c oxidase and restoring its function: red light therapy and methylene blue.

Nitric Oxide Promotes Tumor Growth and Angiogenesis

When metabolism within a cell fails, free radical electrons begin escaping from the respiratory chain, causing damage to the interior contents of the cell, including the mitochondria. This explains why higher levels of reactive oxygen species (free radicals) can be found in Cancer cells and why restoring metabolic function can significantly lower the level of reactive oxygen species generated by cells.

When mitochondria become injured and dysfunctional, they require repair or replacement. Cells become cancerous because their cellular machinery required to produce energy oxidatively becomes damaged, and no other choice exists but to revert to the primitive glycolytic metabolic phenotype of a single-celled organism. It's like firing up a small backup generator to provide electricity for your home.

Despite this, the Cancer industry and governments maintain that a Cancer cell has undergone a Frankenstein-like genetic mutation and suddenly has a thirst for blood – an amazing yet dangerous fairy tale.

My main point here is that Cancer cells *are injured cells* and the breakdown of cellular respiration itself is one way to cause that injury, which is where nitric oxide comes into play.

Anytime a tissue has been injured, nitric oxide and other growth factors are released to signal cells to grow and divide to replace damaged tissue. In an individual with Cancer, tumor cells also receive the message to grow and divide, which is why nitric oxide is a well-known promoter of tumor progression, including angiogenesis—the formation of new vasculature in the area surrounding a tumor.[126]

Nitric Oxide Promotes Cancer Metastasis

Cancer metastasis occurs when a Cancer cell breaks free from a tumor and spreads to another part of the body. Cancer metastasis is the prime cause of death for 90% of Cancer patients.[127]

In Cancer metastasis, after a Cancer cell has escaped from the initial tumor, nitric oxide triggers the adhesion of circulating tumor cells onto body tissues, which is the first step in new tumor formation.[128]

If nitric oxide is such a strong promoter of Cancer, then we should expect any substance that can reduce the concentration or actions of nitric oxide to be beneficial in Cancer. Can methylene blue restore defective mitochondrial function in Cancer?

Methylene Blue Therapy for Cancer

What could be more promising for Cancer than a substance that specifically seeks out and corrects metabolic defects first before anything else? Research on methylene blue for Cancer is surprisingly abundant, dating back almost 100 years, and shows us that methylene blue can rapidly oxygenate Cancer cells and tumors.

The effects of methylene blue on mitochondrial respiration of normal cells are very different than on tumor cells. E.S. Guzman Barron from Johns Hopkins University in Baltimore, Maryland published a study in 1930 in which he states "…methylene blue exerts its catalytic power only on cells or tissues possessing aerobic glycolysis."[129] This remarkable finding means that methylene blue selectively seeks out Cancerous tumor cells and boosts their metabolism while leaving healthy cells unaffected. The closer a cell is to having a tumor cell phenotype, the more potential benefit methylene blue can have.

The potential benefits of methylene blue to tumor cells include increased oxygen consumption and ATP energy generation. "Different kinds of tumors were used in these experiments: human carcinoma, rat sarcoma, rat adenocarcinoma, and Rous chicken sarcoma with the same results, namely that there is a definite increase in the oxygen consumption of these tissues in the presence of methylene blue," continued Barron, who suggested that growing tumor cell cultures for several generations in a medium containing methylene blue dye might *permanently* change those Cancer cells back into normal tissue.

The aerobic glycolysis seen in Cancer cells tells us they are not receiving everything they need to metabolize properly. Methylene blue can help by correcting metabolic defects at complexes I-IV. Red light therapy is another way to restore mitochondrial respiration within tumor cells rapidly. The combination of light therapy with methylene blue for Cancer, called photodynamic therapy, has become one of the most promising and popular research subjects in recent decades.

Photodynamic Therapy for Cancer

Photodynamic therapy involves the use of light therapy in combination with a 'photosensitizer,' one of which can be methylene blue. Red light therapy and methylene blue share a common mechanism of enhancement of mitochondrial respiration, which protects and restores respiration in cells, organs, and body systems. Photodynamic therapy is well known to kill many types of bacteria, parasites, fungi, viruses, and other microorganisms; it has been reported to cause "massive cell death of tumor cells."[130]

Over the past few decades, research publications on photodynamic therapy for Cancer have shot through the roof.

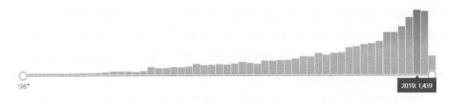

**Photodynamic Therapy for Cancer research publications, 1967-2021.
Source: PubMed**

"Defects in cytochrome c oxidase expression induce a metabolic shift to glycolysis and carcinogenesis," wrote scientists from the University of Pennsylvania in 2015.[131] Red light can photodissociate nitric oxide from cytochrome c oxidase enzymes and upregulate their activity, effectively restoring a Cancer cell back to a normal cell.[132]

While red light therapy primarily targets complex IV, methylene blue exerts its effects on every single complex in the respiratory chain I-IV, which is why combining red light therapy and methylene blue dye therapy are so synergistic and powerful. Drinking water or juice containing a few drops of methylene blue then sitting underneath red light allows you to receive one of the most potent metabolic treatment protocols ever devised. This explains the excitement and skyrocketing publication activity of photodynamic therapy for Cancer among the scientific community in recent years.

Brazilian scientists Tardivo, Giglio, Santos de Oliveira, and their colleagues in Sao Paulo summed up the potential of methylene blue for Cancer when they wrote, "MB has the potential to treat a variety of cancerous and non-cancerous diseases, with low toxicity and no side effects."[133]

The Methylene Blue Battery

After ingesting methylene blue and then urinating into the toilet a few hours later, medicine has been added to the municipal water supply that will help protect people and wildlife from the many highly toxic contaminants typically found in city water, including pharmaceutical drugs, hormones, herbicides and pesticides, rocket fuel, chlorine, arsenic, lead, fluoride, and other poisons.

The same cannot be said for the industrial use of methylene blue. In textile mills using methylene blue to dye fabric, wastewater with high concentrations of methylene blue are created and often added to the environment. Like water, salt, sunlight, or virtually anything else in excess, methylene blue in excess can be detrimental to humans, animals, and the environment. That's why a group of environmentally conscious scientists thought of a brilliant strategy to repurpose the methylene blue-rich wastewater produced by textile mills: a methylene blue battery.

"There's been a lot of work done on ways to sequester methylene blue out of water, but the problem with a lot of these methods is that they're expensive and generate other kinds of waste products," said lead author Anjula Kosswattaarachchi from The State University of New York. "But what if instead of just cleaning the water up, we could find a new way to use it? That's what really motivated this project," continued Anjula.

In 2018, Anjula and Professor Timothy R. Cook decided to create two battery prototypes using methylene blue to see if it would work.[1] Cook and Kosswattaarachchi discovered that when dissolved in water, methylene blue is very efficient at storing energy and then releasing it on cue. In fact, their methylene blue battery might be the most efficient non-toxic battery this world has ever seen.

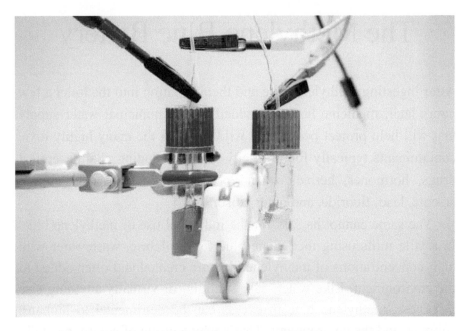

**The methylene blue (MB) battery contains MB solution (left side)
and a colorless solution of leuco methylene blue (right),
which is methylene blue with added electrons.
Photo credit: Meredith Forrest Kulwicki/University at Buffalo**

The first methylene blue battery the team created operated at near-perfect efficiency. After charging and draining the battery 50 times, almost 100% of the electrical energy they put in, they got back out. However, over time, the battery's capacity for energy storage began to drop as molecules of methylene blue became trapped in a membrane critical to the device's function.

To solve this, they created a second prototype using a different membrane material that would not absorb molecules of methylene blue as the first battery did. This new prototype had all the efficiency of the first battery, and no longer showed any drop in efficiency after 12 cycles of charging and discharging. Problem solved!

The results of their study have established that methylene blue is an exceptional material for liquid batteries. So let it be known!

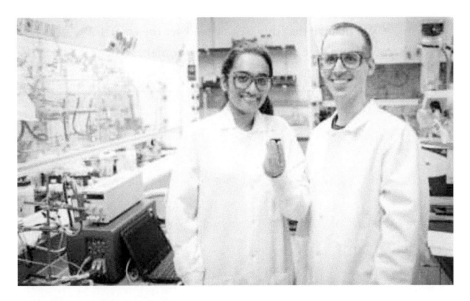

Scientists Anjula Kosswattaarachchi (left), a PhD student in chemistry, and Timothy Cook, an assistant professor of chemistry, exploring whether methylene blue from industrial wastewater can be used to power organic batteries. Photo credit: Meredith Forrest Kulwicki/University at Buffalo

Battery technology on the market today comes with a significant negative environmental impact. Lead-acid batteries contain numerous toxic heavy metals like acid, lead, nickel, cadmium, and mercury, all of which escape into the environment after being used up and disposed. Furthermore, the recent rise in electric cars on the market will eventually result in a mountain of toxic waste from spent batteries if we do nothing to change the underlying technology in the batteries used in these vehicles.

A new battery that's clean and safe for Earth's environment is needed as humanity moves towards living in a way that has a net positive impact on the natural world – and that new battery has been found!

Kosswattaarachchi expressed her hope for a better future based on their breakthrough methylene blue battery:

"We believe that this work could set the stage for
an alternative route for wastewater management,
paving a path to a green-energy storage technology."[2]

Methylene Blue for Dogs, Cats, Cows, Fish and Horses

Fish enthusiasts know how delicate an aquarium environment can be and how quickly an imbalance or the wrong thing in the water can kill the fish. Methylene blue does the opposite, protecting fish from infection and damage caused by chemical contaminants like ammonia and nitrite poisoning. Methylene blue is the first-line defense in aquariums to safely and effectively disinfect water and protect fish from fungal infections, which is a testament to how safe it is.

Methylene blue is currently not approved for veterinary use in the United States or Canada, so there are no veterinary-labeled commercial methylene blue products on the market. This is unfortunate because it appears methylene blue has every bit as much potential for helping our animal friends as it does humans. Virtually every benefit of methylene blue shown in humans was first discovered in studies on rats or other animals before being validated in human clinical trials.

Although more methylene blue animal experiments showing safety and efficacy would be helpful for it to receive approval as veterinary medicine, methylene blue is still often used by veterinarians to treat methemoglobinemia in various species of animals, including cattle, goats, sheet, cats, dogs, horses, etc.[1] Scientific research shows us some of the many other things methylene blue can do for animals. In cows, for example, methylene blue inhibits the parasite Neospora caninum, which has been strongly associated with reproductive problems.[2] Cows are sometimes poisoned with nitrates through fertilizer contamination in their water supply. A 1983 study published in *The Veterinary Record* showed that treatment with methylene blue (1mg/kg) was an effective antidote.[3] Another issue cows can face is infected sole ulcers. In a 2018 case report on a cow suffering from an infected sole ulcer, photodynamic therapy improved the condition in one week, and complete healing was achieved in 57 days.[4]

But you probably don't own a cow or care about how to heal them, so how about the use of methylene blue for the two most common house pets: dogs and cats? A male mixed breed dog with lethargy, exercise intolerance, and aggression when touched on its head was found to have methemoglobinemia and treated using methylene blue in a 2017 study by researchers at the University of Pennsylvania. "The methemoglobinemia and associated clinical signs resolved after administration of methylene blue (1 mg/kg) IV, and the dog was discharged," wrote scientists. After 11 days, the symptoms returned, and a maintenance dose of 1.5mg/kg (initially daily, then every other day) normalized both the dog's symptoms and methemoglobin concentrations.[5]

In cats, it's been claimed that methylene blue is contraindicated and can cause Heinz body (HB) hemolytic anemia. So, a group of scientists from Kansas State University in Manhattan tested that theory while simultaneously examining the efficacy and safety of methylene blue for methemoglobinemia in cats. The study reports that one IV dose (1.5mg/kg) of methylene blue "sufficiently and rapidly reversed MTHB [methemoglobinemia] in the cats," with no increase in Heinz body-containing red blood cells. However, two doses without or after sodium nitrite "significantly increased the frequency of circulating HB-containing red blood cells," leading the researchers to conclude that "pre-exposure to sodium nitrite potentiated the HB-inducing effect of two doses of MB." The important lesson here is that one dose was reported safe, and two doses had some negative side effects, making the case that low doses are overall better.[6]

As you can see, methylene blue could be a useful medicine for your house pets. However, would I recommend people start feeding their dogs and cats a few drops of methylene blue as a preventative or medicine? I think in time, methylene blue will become known as one of the safest and most effective medicines for humans and other creatures for many conditions. I don't want anybody blaming me for the death of their pets after feeding them an entire bottle of methylene blue, so no, I don't recommend it. I recommend that *if* you choose to give methylene blue to your pets, take complete responsibility for your actions and their consequences.

Safety, Dose, & Where to Get Methylene Blue?

Methylene blue is sold in crystalline powder form and as a liquid that can easily be added to drinks with a dropper and consumed orally.

When supplementing methylene blue, you can expect aquamarine-colored urine between 4 and 12 hours after consumption. This is of particular importance for men, who will need to apply added focus while urinating so as not to paint the walls or floor. I'm only half-joking about that.

1. High vs. Low Dose?

Methylene blue exhibits very different effects at low doses than it does at high doses. They call this a 'hormetic dose response,' where the effects of a low dose are the opposite than at a high dose.

"Methylene blue is a safe drug when used in therapeutic doses (<2mg/kg). But it can cause toxicity in high doses," wrote Prashant R. Ginimuge and S.D. Jyothi from the Belgaum Institute of Medical Sciences in Karnataka, India.[1]

At low doses, methylene blue acts as an antioxidant within mitochondria by improving the efficiency of electron transfer between the four complexes within the mitochondrial electron transport chain. As a result, fewer superoxide radicals are generated during the process of oxidative phosphorylation. Methylene blue can also prevent electron leakage caused by anything that inhibits mitochondrial function, like environmental chemicals. It improves the metabolic rate by bypassing blocked points of electron flow during mitochondrial respiration.[2]

At high doses, methylene blue can actually have the opposite effect, promoting free radical production and oxidative stress in the body by "stealing" electrons from the electron transport chain complexes, acting as a pro-oxidant, and causing an increase in reactive oxygen species.[2] Interestingly, Vitamin B3 (niacinamide) has been shown to reduce the cytotoxic effects of high doses of methylene blue.[3] Overall, the potential increase in oxidative stress that high doses of methylene blue can cause adds to the case that low doses are better than higher ones. And that case is further strengthened by the potential for impurities in the methylene blue itself.

Methylene Blue Grades: Beware of Impurities!

Adverse effects of methylene blue can come from chemical impurities, so it's important to use only pharmaceutical-grade methylene blue. Don't be afraid to ask for a lab analysis to confirm the purity of the product when buying. At low doses, these contaminants are not that big of a problem. But higher doses can result in the accumulation of toxins in your cells, so it's critical to understand the different grades of methylene blue on the market.

There are three different grades of methylene blue:

1. **Industrial grade** – used to dye fabric
2. **Chemical grade** – used in laboratory experiments
3. **Pharmaceutical grade** – used to treat methemoglobinemia, urinary tract infections, overdoses, and considered safe for human use

According to Sigma Chemical Company in St Louis, Missouri, industrial-grade or chemical-grade methylene blue sold as a dye or stain can consist of 8-11% or more of various contaminants, like arsenic, aluminum, cadmium, mercury, and lead, and should not be administered to humans or animals.[4]

Researchers from the University of Texas inform us that even pharmaceutical (USP) grade methylene blue can contain impurities, making the case for taking low doses of methylene blue even more compelling. "At low doses, the presence of contaminants is not of great concern, but at higher doses, non-specific effects due to accumulation of various toxic and bioactive substances are possible."[4]

For anybody looking to try methylene, it's imperative that you purchase and use only pharmaceutical grade methylene blue – never chemical or industrial grade.

Pharmaceutical grade methylene blue receives its certification by meeting a strict set of manufacturing protocols and must exceed 99% purity and not contain any fillers, binders, or other inactive ingredients. Choosing a pharmaceutical-grade supplement is the only way to know for certain that you're using the highest, purest, and most bioavailable form of methylene blue possible.

Potential Drug Reactions with Methylene Blue

For those who suffer from depression and are intrigued by the potential of using methylene blue instead of toxic and side-effect-laden SSRI drugs, it's important to note that some published case studies have found negative drug reactions between SSRI psychiatric drugs and methylene blue. After intravenous infusion of higher doses of methylene blue, some patients developed "an acute confusional state" and other symptoms consistent with serotonin syndrome.[5]

Does this mean that someone on SSRIs has no hope of switching to methylene blue? Absolutely not. It just means that it's probably best to wean off the drug for a while before making the switch.

Something that might also help make the transition is red light therapy. A study from Harvard found that one single treatment of red light therapy directly against the forehead resulted in long-lasting beneficial effects on both anxiety and depression scores. Talk to your doctor first before you do anything, and be sure to bring her a copy of this book to read.

2. The Most Effective Dose?

Since methylene blue is only FDA-approved for methemoglobinemia, safe and effective doses for other conditions have not yet been established. However, there is no shortage of clinical studies from which we can establish a dose that appears to be safe and effective.

A methylene blue dose commonly used in human clinical trials is 2mg/kg, which rarely causes side effects. Side effects are even rarer at a dose of 1mg/kg.[6]

When doses above 2mg/kg are taken, methylene blue begins to function as a Monoamine Oxidase Inhibitor (MAOI), which increases the action of serotonin and can lead to serotonin syndrome other side effects, including:[7]

- Shortness of breath

- Chest pain

- Dizziness

- Headache

- Sweating

- Confusion

- Increased heart rate

- Abnormal skin sensations (tingling, chilling, burning, numbness)

- Restlessness

- Nausea

When doctors administer methylene blue to patients intravenously for treating methemoglobinemia, they use a dose of 1-2mg/kg.[7]

The dose of methylene blue needed for nitric oxide inhibition and to scavenge free-floating nitric oxide in the blood is surprisingly small. Dr. Raymond Peat has said that 1 to 2mg of methylene blue per day is probably plenty, but for most conditions studied in this book, like Alzheimer's, depression, Cancer, and others, an oral daily dose in the range of 10 to 60mg in divided doses seems to be the ideal.

The dose that appears the most beneficial ranges from 10mg per day all the way up to 2mg/kg methylene blue per day in divided doses.

How Do I Take Methylene Blue?

Aside from life-threatening or emergency situations, like drug overdose or chemical poisoning (methemoglobinemia), where 1-2mg/kg infusions are administered in hospital emergency rooms, I recommend beginning methylene blue therapy with a 10mg per day dose, regardless of your bodyweight.

With a 1% methylene blue solution (like the one I recommend at the end of this book), each drop contains 0.5mg of methylene blue, which means to achieve a 10 mg dose you'll need 20 drops of methylene blue.

Begin by adding 10 drops (5mg) to a glass of water or juice and drinking it in the morning, and 10 drops (5mg) to a glass or water or juice and drinking it in the evening before bed. Try this for 1 week, and if it's well tolerated and you want more, increase your dose to 20mg/day.

For a 20mg/day dose, add 20 drops (10mg) to a glass of water or juice and drink in the morning and 20 drops (10mg) to a glass of water or juice and drink in the evening before bed.

At the end of the second week, if you want to further increase your methylene blue dose, try increasing it to 30mg/day. Continue this pattern until you've reached your desired dose.

	Total Daily Dose	Morning	Evening
Week 1	10mg	10 drops (5mg)	10 drops (5mg)
Week 2	20mg	20 drops (10mg)	20 drops (10mg)
Week 3	30mg	30 drops (15mg)	30 drops (15mg)

Our world is undeniably toxic, and between the chemicals we're exposed to in food, water, air, personal care products, and the 24/7 radiation from cell phones, cell phone towers, and wireless routers, I consume and recommend 10mg methylene blue daily (even in healthy individuals) in a glass of orange juice to compensate for our imperfect environment.

One thing you'll notice, even at the very low dose range of 10 mg, is that your teeth and mouth may be temporarily colored blue. Do not be alarmed. This is normal and to be expected when using methylene blue. The blue color will disappear once your body uses it. If you find it to be problematic, try taking methylene blue before bed only so your body has adequate time to use it while you sleep.

For those interested in taking doses ranging from 0.5mg/kg to 2.0mg/kg – the doses found safe and effective in clinical studies – I've created a chart for you below so you can determine the correct dose for your bodyweight without having to get out your calculator. First, find your approximate bodyweight in the left hand column, and then look to the right to see the corresponding dose and number of drops you'll need to take per day.

Methylene Blue Doses (1% Solution)			
Bodyweight	0.5 mg/kg	1 mg/kg	2 mg/kg
50kg/110lbs	25mg dose (50 drops/day)	50mg dose (100 drops/day)	100mg dose (200 drops/day)
55kg/121lbs	27.5mg dose (55 drops/day)	55mg dose (110 drops/day)	110mg dose (220 drops/day)
60kg/132lbs	30mg dose (60 drops/day)	60mg dose (120 drops/day)	120mg dose (240 drops/day)
65kg/143lbs	32.5mg dose (65 drops/day)	65mg dose (130 drops/day)	130mg dose (260 drops/day)
70kg/154lbs	35mg dose (70 drops/day)	70mg dose (140 drops/day)	140mg dose (280 drops/day)
75kg/165lbs	37.5mg dose (75 drops/day)	75mg dose (150 drops/day)	150mg dose (300 drops/day)
80kg/176lbs	40mg dose (80 drops/day)	80mg dose (160 drops/day)	160mg dose (320 drops/day)
85kg/187lbs	42.5mg dose (85 drops/day)	85mg dose (170 drops/day)	170mg dose (340 drops/day)

90kg/198lbs	45mg dose (90 drops/day)	90mg dose (180 drops/day)	180mg dose (360 drops/day)
95kg/209lbs	47.5mg dose (95 drops/day)	95mg dose (190 drops/day)	190mg dose (380 drops/day)
100kg/220lbs	50mg dose (100 drops/day)	100mg dose (200 drops/day)	200mg dose (400 drops/day)

At higher doses, you may find that the taste of your methylene blue drink becomes less palatable. If that's the case, don't be afraid to increase the number of doses per day to 3, 4, 5, or even more in order to reduce the quantity of methylene blue in each drink. I hope you found this information helpful.

Shelf-Life

Stamped on a bottle of methylene blue I recently purchased was a "best before" date of five years. Curious about what happens at that 5-year point, I asked a friend who is a chemist involved in synthesizing methylene blue: "Does methylene blue *actually* expire and go bad, or is that expiry date just to cover your ass?"

I take no liability whatsoever for anyone using methylene blue beyond the expiry date marked on the bottle, and neither does my friend the chemist, but his response was: Methylene blue is *extremely* stable, and "as long as you store it in a dark bottle and out of sunlight, it'll last virtually forever."

General Safety Guidelines

Although side effects at low doses are rare, I've put together some general guidelines for maximizing the safety of using methylene blue, most of which are common sense.[8]

- Methylene blue should not be taken with SSRI medication.

- Methylene blue should not be given to babies.

- Do not use methylene blue if you are pregnant or breast feeding.

Where to get Methylene Blue?

If you're going to take methylene blue, it's important to remember to only buy pharmaceutical-grade products to avoid ingesting impurities like toxic heavy metals.

In preparation for the launch of this book, I found a company that manufactures pure pharmaceutical-grade methylene blue in the United States. I phoned and asked if they would be interested in partnering and providing a discount code to readers of this book so that I can send people to them to buy methylene blue.

They accepted my offer and now I've got a discount code for 10% off USP grade methylene blue for you. If you buy from them, not only are you getting a premium quality product, but you're buying a product that is actually made in the USA rather than in China for once, which is something to feel good about.

Your discount code and a link to the product can be found at the end of this book.

Conclusion

In his article "Truth in Basic Biomedical Science Will Set Future Mankind Free," Dr. Gilbert Ling wrote that major scientific innovations "grow only in the exceptionally fertile minds of men and women, who have fully mastered the underlying basic sciences. To waken their interest in science at an early critical age and to nurture and enhance that interest afterward, good textbooks at all levels of education that accurately portray the relevant up-to-date knowledge are vital. As of now, the field of science that offers by far the greatest promise for the future of humanity is the science of life at the most basic cell and below-cell level."

The purpose of this book is to serve as the "textbook" that Ling mentioned, except to take it a couple of steps further by transferring the major breakthroughs and scientific discoveries out of the realm of academia and directly into the hands of the public who need it.

"Health is the greatest of human blessings."

These were the words of the founder of modern medicine and Greek physician Hippocrates, born in 460BC. Still true today, health is the foundation for a sane, rational, and righteous life. Groups of healthy people and families are the foundations for a sane, rational and righteous society.

The greatest obstacle preventing humanity from thriving as we move forward through time is the existing for-profit medical paradigm, which is based on the belief that diseases are genetically determined and incurable. If diseases are all genetic in origin and incurable, then treating symptoms is the best we can do. But a steady stream of groundbreaking discoveries made by scientists worldwide over the preceding centuries has made it clear that genetic mutations are symptoms of disease rather than causes, all diseases are metabolic in origin, and metabolic defects can be corrected.

Humanity's Transition from Genetic to Metabolic Medicine

According to the modern medical establishment, there are over 32,000 different diseases in existence today, all with unique pathologies and genetic mutations. The purpose of this artificial complexity is not only to sell more drugs, but to generate in the public a feeling of overwhelm, helplessness, and despair in regards to ever understanding what disease is and how to heal it on their own – making them dependent on medical doctors. But the joke is on us: Medical doctors are taught nothing about what disease is and how it manifests in the body – only how to fatten the pockets of large drug company CEOs through the prescription of expensive and mostly-toxic drugs and surgeries. The French philosopher Voltaire said it best:

"Doctors put drugs of which they know little into bodies of which they know less for diseases of which they know nothing at all."

The groundbreaking 2003 study by Dr. Gary Null and his team of scientists called *Death By Medicine* revealed to us an ugly, dark, yet important truth: modern medicine is *literally* the number one cause of death in the United States (and probably the entire world today). The existing genetic paradigm of disease has been a complete and utter failure.

As the medical establishment continues its forward march of destruction–pretending knives, poison pills, and other anti-metabolic stress factors like nitric oxide, estrogen, serotonin are therapeutic for people while performing countless unnecessary procedures, inducing unnecessary suffering and leaving many victims in its wake – a new paradigm is taking shape.

Around 2500 years ago, Hippocrates wrote, "It's far more important to know what person the disease has than what disease the person has," and I think it's time we listen. There is only one disease, and that disease is a malfunctioning cell.

The worldwide revolution currently underway in medicine involves a shift from therapies targeting symptoms and mutated genes to a new class of therapies that directly target the metabolic defects underlying disease.

Targeting Metabolic Dysfunction

The bioenergetic state of cells in our body is paramount when it comes to our overall level of health. If our cellular mitochondria are metabolizing properly, oxygen is being used to manufacture energy and highly valuable carbon dioxide molecules, which dilate blood vessels and drive oxygen into cells. When cellular mitochondria become compromised by nutritional deficiencies or toxic chemical exposure, energy production by cells slows, and it's this breakdown of mitochondrial energy production that underlies all the unwanted symptoms characteristic of disease.

Seemingly miraculous healing has occurred in many people using the metabolic medicine red light therapy (you can read many of the testimonials in my book *Red Light Therapy: Miracle Medicine*). The action of red light on the complex IV cytochrome c oxidase enzyme within the mitochondria of cells is responsible for this healing. When red light is shone onto cells, this enzyme absorbs the light, resulting in increased manufacture of cellular ATP energy.

If red light therapy can bestow such remarkable benefit from its actions on complex IV within mitochondria, just imagine what a medicine that can bridge defects in complexes I, II, III, *and* IV within mitochondria could do. That medicine is methylene blue.

Methylene blue has the power to not only restore mitochondrial function in some of the most debilitating diseases we see so commonly in our world today but also has the power to debunk mistaken and dangerous cultural beliefs.

The widespread cultural belief that nitric oxide is a vasodilator with therapeutic effects *is wrong* – and methylene blue proves it. The misuse of nitric oxide agonists like Viagra in medicine, including on pregnant women, is a source of unnecessary suffering and arguably murder that must stop. The hypothesis that nitric oxide is the primary cause of aging in every cell and tissue of the body is probably true. The inexpensive drug methylene blue, a nitric oxide antagonist, has proven itself useful for remedying mitochondrial dysfunction perhaps better than any other known medicine.

Doctor Yourself

Nobody can know you, or what you need to heal, more than yourself, which is probably why Hippocrates wrote,

---

"If you are not your own doctor, you are a fool."

He was right when he said it back then, and today it's even more true. Never before in history have metabolic therapies like methylene blue, red light therapy, balneotherapy, sodium bicarbonate, carbon dioxide, aspirin, niacinamide, pregnenolone, progesterone, DHEA and thyroid been more inexpensive or easily obtainable.

The answers are right before our eyes. The seeds of truth needed to set future mankind free – the major scientific innovations that "grow only in the exceptionally fertile minds of men and women, who have fully mastered the underlying basic sciences," as Ling put it – have now been planted. Go forth and use them to improve yourself and spread the news to the good people around you.

Bonus: The Blue Bottle Experiment

Now that you've finished reading this book, it's time for a metaphorical 'champagne popping' to celebrate everything methylene blue has to offer. The Blue Bottle Experiment is a classic chemistry experiment involving a methylene blue solution that you can use to impress all your friends and family.

High school chemistry teachers often do The Blue Bottle Experiment to demonstrate oxidation and reduction reactions to students. In the experiment, a methylene blue solution is "magically" transformed from blue to colourless, and then back again by shaking it. Of course, it's not magic at all; it just takes a little understanding of chemistry to explain this fascinating phenomenon.

How it Works

Methylene blue is a crystalline substance that yields a blue liquid when dissolved in water. When sugar is added to that water, it reacts with the methylene blue and turns the solution colorless. And when you shake the colorless liquid, the methylene blue reacts with oxygen introduced by the shaking, restoring the blue color.

The color change occurs because methylene blue exists in two forms. The first is a reduced form, which is colorless, and the other is an oxidized form, which is the classic blue color. The cycling between oxidized and reduced forms makes methylene blue *a redox agent* and explains how it helps prevent oxidant production within cellular mitochondria.

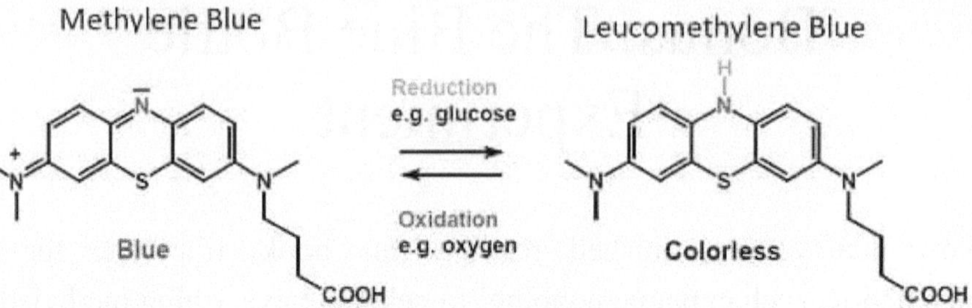

Methylene Blue   Leucomethylene Blue

Reduction
e.g. glucose

Oxidation
e.g. oxygen

Blue   Colorless

The two forms of methylene blue. Image source: Genelink.com

This flip-flop from colored liquid to clear liquid can be performed a number of times in this experiment until either the oxygen or the glucose in the bottle are fully consumed. Of course, you can add additional oxygen by uncapping the liquid for a few moments to let fresh air into the bottle. To continue the experiment indefinitely, add more glucose to the liquid.

Now that you have a basic understanding of how it all works, here's what you need to know to perform the experiment yourself.

Materials needed:

- Glucose
- 1% methylene blue solution
- Potassium hydroxide
- Distilled water
- 500mL flask with stopper
- 500mL graduated cylinder
- 2 x weighing dishes

Preparation:

To prepare your "blue bottle" solution,

1. Begin by adding 300mL of distilled water to your 500mL flask.

2. Add 8 grams of potassium hydroxide to the water, and stir until the solid is dissolved.
3. Add 10 grams of glucose and a few drops of methylene blue to that same flask and fill the remainder with water until it reaches the 500mL mark.
4. Once complete, cap the flask with your stopper and mix thoroughly.

Procedure:

Once the solution is prepared, you can either transfer it to a water bottle and cap the lid or leave it in the 500mL flask and cap it with a stopper.

Whichever vessel you choose, set the bottle down and let it rest undisturbed for a few minutes until the solution becomes colorless.

Now your 'magic' blue bottle demonstration can begin! Show everybody your bottle of clear "water," and then *gently* shake it and watch it turn blue. Voila! The universe just folded inside out for everybody watching.

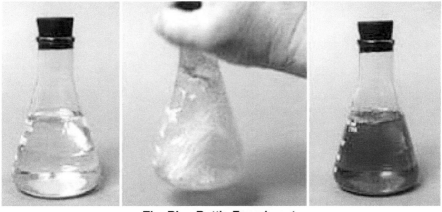

The Blue Bottle Experiment.
Image source: University of Wisconsin Department of Chemistry

Once the solution inside your bottle is entirely blue, put it down and let it rest until the liquid becomes clear once again. You can repeat this process several times for about 15 minutes. At some point, you will need to remove the cap to re-introduce more oxygen into your bottle or add more glucose.

Disposal:

After you're done with the experiment, flush the solution down the drain and feel good that you've added something beneficial to the water supply that will protect all life everywhere.

The Blue Bottle Experiment is a simple and timeless experiment that can be done by pretty much anyone to illustrate the reduction and oxidation properties of methylene blue or to get children interested in science.

To all the students out there: Be sure to ask your chemistry teacher to do The Blue Bottle Experiment for you in class at least once a week.

About the Author

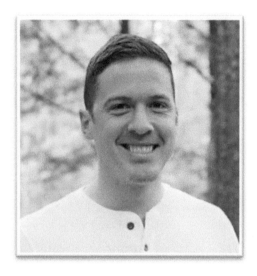

MARK SLOAN has written over 300 articles and is the author of *The Cancer Industry, Cancer: The Metabolic Disease Unravelled* and the 6x international #1 bestseller *Red Light Therapy: Miracle Medicine*. Mark lives in Ontario, Canada, and his goal is to build his home from scratch, entirely off grid, then start a family and live a self-sufficient, resilient, and responsible life as God had intended. Mark is passionate about learning, and his ultimate goal in life is to reduce the unnecessary suffering in this world and to make a better place for every human being alive and for future generations.

Please Review This!

I hope you enjoyed this book and found the information valuable. Above all, I hope it gives you hope for a brighter future.

If this book helped or entertained you in any way, all I ask in return is that you take a moment to write an honest, sincere review of this book on Amazon. It will only take a few minutes, and it will help me out more than you can imagine.

To leave a review, search "Methylene blue Mark Sloan" on Amazon to find the book page or visit the following link, then scroll down and write a couple of quick sentences:
https://www.amazon.com/dp/177723963X

More #1 Bestselling Books By The Author

- The Cancer Industry
- Cancer: The Metabolic Disease Unravelled
- Red Light Therapy: Miracle Medicine
- The Ultimate Guide to Methylene Blue: Remarkable Hope for
- Bath Bombs & Balneotherapy
- And more!

Checkout all of Mark Sloan's books by visiting the following link:

https://endalldisease.com/books

A Free Gift From the Author

Find out which pharmaceutical grade methylene blue I use, and get a discount code for 10% off. Click the link below to find out, <u>absolutely FREE!</u>

- ✓ Pharmaceutical (USP) Grade
- ✓ Made in the United States
- ✓ Lab Tested for Purity
- ✓ 10% Off Discount Code

Visit:
EndAllDisease.com/mb

REFERENCES

Introduction

[1] Jaffey JA, Harmon MR, Villani NA, et al. Long-term treatment with methylene blue in a dog with hereditary methemoglobinemia caused by cytochrome b5 reductase deficiency. J Vet Intern Med. 2017;31(6):1860-1865.
https://www.ncbi.nlm.nih.gov/pmc/articles/PMC5697180

2 World Health Organization Model List of Essential Medicines. 2019. Source:
https://apps.who.int/iris/bitstream/handle/10665/325771/WHO-MVP-EMP-IAU-2019.06-eng.pdf

Nitric Oxide: Miracle Molecule or Aging Accelerant?

1 Culotta E, Koshland DE. NO news is good news. Science. 1992;258(5090):1862-1865. https://science.sciencemag.org/content/258/5090/1862

2 Oyeyipo IP, Raji Y, Bolarinwa AF. Ng-nitro-l-arginine methyl ester protects against hormonal imbalances associated with nicotine administration in male rats. N Am J Med Sci. 2015;7(2):59-64.
https://www.ncbi.nlm.nih.gov/pmc/articles/PMC4358050

3 Cotter G, Kaluski E, Milo O, et al. Lincs: l-name (A no synthase inhibitor) in the treatment of refractory cardiogenic shock: a prospective randomized study. European Heart Journal. 2003;24(14):1287-1295.
https://academic.oup.com/eurheartj/article/24/14/1287/501770

4 Pershing NLK, Yang C-FJ, Xu M, Counter CM. Treatment with the nitric oxide synthase inhibitor L-NAME provides a survival advantage in a mouse model of Kras mutation-positive, non-small cell lung cancer. Oncotarget. 2016;7(27):42385-42392.
https://www.ncbi.nlm.nih.gov/pmc/articles/PMC5173142

5 Lampson BL, Kendall SD, Ancrile BB, et al. Targeting eNOS in pancreatic cancer. Cancer Res. 2012;72(17):4472-4482. https://pubmed.ncbi.nlm.nih.gov/22738914

[6] Beckman KB, Ames BN. The free radical theory of aging matures. Physiological Reviews. 1998;78(2):547-581.
https://journals.physiology.org/doi/full/10.1152/physrev.1998.78.2.547

[7] Burning Question: Can you have too many antioxidants? ABC Health & Wellbeing. 2017. Olivia Willis. Source: https://www.abc.net.au/news/health/2017-04-21/can-you-have-too-many-antioxidants/8457336

[8] Wang X, Wu L, Aouffen M, Mateescu M-A, Nadeau R, Wang R. Novel cardiac protective effects of urea: from shark to rat. Br J Pharmacol. 1999;128(7):1477-1484. https://www.ncbi.nlm.nih.gov/pmc/articles/PMC1571786

[9] Choi SYC, Collins CC, Gout PW, Wang Y. Cancer-generated lactic acid: a regulatory, immunosuppressive metabolite? J Pathol. 2013;230(4):350-355. https://www.ncbi.nlm.nih.gov/pmc/articles/PMC3757307

[10] Wahl P, Zinner C, Achtzehn S, Bloch W, Mester J. Effect of high- and low-intensity exercise and metabolic acidosis on levels of GH, IGF-I, IGFBP-3 and cortisol. Growth Horm IGF Res. 2010;20(5):380-385. https://pubmed.ncbi.nlm.nih.gov/20801067

[11] Dhup S, Dadhich RK, Porporato PE, Sonveaux P. Multiple biological activities of lactic acid in cancer: influences on tumor growth, angiogenesis and metastasis. Curr Pharm Des. 2012;18(10):1319-1330. https://pubmed.ncbi.nlm.nih.gov/22360558

[12] Oyeyipo IP, Raji Y, Bolarinwa AF. Ng-nitro-l-arginine methyl ester protects against hormonal imbalances associated with nicotine administration in male rats. N Am J Med Sci. 2015;7(2):59-64. https://www.ncbi.nlm.nih.gov/pmc/articles/PMC4358050

[13] Panesar NS, Chan KW. Decreased steroid hormone synthesis from inorganic nitrite and nitrate: studies in vitro and in vivo. Toxicol Appl Pharmacol. 2000;169(3):222-230. https://pubmed.ncbi.nlm.nih.gov/11133344

[14] Morgan JC, Alhatou M, Oberlies J, Johnston KC. Transient ischemic attack and stroke associated with sildenafil (Viagra) use. *Neurology*. 2001;57(9):1730-1731. https://n.neurology.org/content/57/9/1730.short

[15] Lowe G, Costabile RA. 10-Year analysis of adverse event reports to the Food and Drug Administration for phosphodiesterase type-5 inhibitors. J Sex Med. 2012;9(1):265-270. https://pubmed.ncbi.nlm.nih.gov/22023666

[16] Calabrese V, Scapagnini G, Ravagna A, et al. Nitric oxide synthase is present in the cerebrospinal fluid of patients with active multiple sclerosis and is associated with increases in cerebrospinal fluid protein nitrotyrosine and S-nitrosothiols and with changes in glutathione levels. J Neurosci Res. 2002;70(4):580-587. https://pubmed.ncbi.nlm.nih.gov/12404512

[17] Togo T, Katsuse O, Iseki E. Nitric oxide pathways in Alzheimer's disease and other neurodegenerative dementias. Neurol Res. 2004;26(5):563-566. https://pubmed.ncbi.nlm.nih.gov/15265275

[18] Li W-Q, Qureshi AA, Robinson KC, Han J. Sildenafil use and increased risk of incident melanoma in US men: a prospective cohort study. JAMA Intern Med. 2014;174(6):964-970. https://pubmed.ncbi.nlm.nih.gov/24710960

[19] Sharma S, Panda S, Sharma S, Singh SK, Seth A, Gupta N. Prolonged priapism following single dose administration of sildenafil: A rare case report. Urology Annals. 2009;1(2):67.
https://www.urologyannals.com/article.asp?issn=0974-7796;year=2009;volume=1;issue=2;spage=67;epage=68;aulast=Sharma

[20] Hard luck – Viagra can cause impotence. Independent. 1999. Jeremy Laurance. Source: https://www.independent.co.uk/news/hard-luck-viagra-can-cause-impotence-1076636.html

[21] Man's penis amputated after Viagra overdose. Independent. 2013. Nick Renaud-Komiya. Source: https://www.independent.co.uk/news/world/americas/man-s-penis-amputated-after-viagra-overdose-8835146.html

[22] Nisoli E, Carruba MO. Nitric oxide and mitochondrial biogenesis. J Cell Sci. 2006;119(Pt 14):2855-2862. https://pubmed.ncbi.nlm.nih.gov/16825426

[23] Chuang I-C, Yang R-C, Chou S-H, et al. Effect of carbon dioxide inhalation on pulmonary hypertension induced by increased blood flow and hypoxia. Kaohsiung J Med Sci. 2011;27(8):336-343. https://pubmed.ncbi.nlm.nih.gov/21802645

[24] Hwang J-H, Kim K-J, Ryu S-J, Lee B-Y. Caffeine prevents LPS-induced inflammatory responses in RAW264.7 cells and zebrafish. Chem Biol Interact. 2016;248:1-7. https://pubmed.ncbi.nlm.nih.gov/26852703

[25] Pels A, Kenny LC, Alfirevic Z, et al. STRIDER (Sildenafil TheRapy in dismal prognosis early onset fetal growth restriction): an international consortium of randomised placebo-controlled trials. BMC Pregnancy Childbirth. 2017;17(1):440. https://pubmed.ncbi.nlm.nih.gov/29282009

[26] How ebola kills you: It's not the virus. NPR. 2014. Michaeleen Doucleff. Source: https://www.npr.org/sections/goatsandsoda/2014/08/26/342451672/how-ebola-kills-you-its-not-the-virus

[27] Sanchez A, Lukwiya M, Bausch D, et al. Analysis of human peripheral blood samples from fatal and nonfatal cases of Ebola (Sudan) hemorrhagic fever: cellular responses,

virus load, and nitric oxide levels. J Virol. 2004;78(19):10370-10377.
https://pubmed.ncbi.nlm.nih.gov/15367603

Gene Therapy Failure & The Future of Medicine

[1] Annadurai K, Danasekaran R, Mani G. Personalized medicine: A paradigm shift towards promising health care. J Pharm Bioallied Sci. 2016;8(1):77-78.
https://www.ncbi.nlm.nih.gov/pmc/articles/PMC4766785

[2] McCAIN J. The future of gene therapy. Biotechnol Healthc. 2005;2(3):52-60.
https://www.ncbi.nlm.nih.gov/pmc/articles/PMC3564347

[3] At $2.1 million, new gene therapy is the most expensive drug ever. NPR. 2019. Rob Stein. Source: https://www.npr.org/sections/health-shots/2019/05/24/725404168/at-2-125-million-new-gene-therapy-is-the-most-expensive-drug-ever

[4] Galzi J-L. [Gene editing in drug discovery and therapeutic innovation]. Med Sci (Paris). 2019;35(4):309-315. https://pubmed.ncbi.nlm.nih.gov/31038108

[5] DNA-editing breakthrough could fix 'broken genes' in the brain, delay ageing and cure incurable diseases. Independent. 2016. Ian Johnston. Source:
https://www.independent.co.uk/news/science/gene-editing-breakthrough-fix-broken-genes-delay-ageing-cure-incurable-diseases-a7421596.html

[6] Yakovlev VA. Role of nitric oxide in the radiation-induced bystander effect. Redox Biol. 2015;6:396-400. https://pubmed.ncbi.nlm.nih.gov/26355395/

[7] Han W, Wu L, Chen S, et al. Constitutive nitric oxide acting as a possible intercellular signaling molecule in the initiation of radiation-induced DNA double strand breaks in non-irradiated bystander cells. Oncogene. 2007;26(16):2330-9.
https://pubmed.ncbi.nlm.nih.gov/17016433/

[8] Xiao L, Liu W, Li J, et al. Irradiated U937 cells trigger inflammatory bystander responses in human umbilical vein endothelial cells through the p38 pathway. Radiat Res. 2014;182(1):111-21. https://www.jstor.org/stable/24545385

[9] Lala PK, Chakraborty C. Role of nitric oxide in carcinogenesis and tumour progression. Lancet Oncol. 2001;2(3):149-56.
https://pubmed.ncbi.nlm.nih.gov/11902565/

[10] Fernàndez-Ruiz I. Gene therapy: No improvement in outcomes with gene therapy for heart failure. Nat Rev Cardiol. 2016;13(3):122-123.
https://pubmed.ncbi.nlm.nih.gov/26843287

[11] Stevens null, Glatstein null. Beware the medical-industrial complex. Oncologist. 1996;1(4):IV-V. https://pubmed.ncbi.nlm.nih.gov/10388005

[12] Longevity Secrets of the Naked Mole Rat. Endalldisease. 2020. Mark Sloan. Source: https://endalldisease.com/longevity-secrets-naked-mole-rat

[13] Nisoli E, Carruba MO. Nitric oxide and mitochondrial biogenesis. Journal of Cell Science. 2006;119(14):2855-2862. https://jcs.biologists.org/content/119/14/2855

[14] DeBerardinis RJ, Thompson CB. Cellular metabolism and disease: what do metabolic outliers teach us? Cell. 2012;148(6):1132-1144. https://www.cell.com/fulltext/S0092-8674(12)00232-2#%20

Meet Methylene Blue

[1] Who we are 1865-1901. BASF. Source: https://www.basf.com/ca/en/who-we-are/history/1865-1901.html

[2] The right chemistry: Methylene blue shakes up the medical world. Montreal Gazette. 2016. Joe Schwarcz. Source: https://montrealgazette.com/opinion/columnists/the-right-chemistry-methylene-blue-shakes-up-the-medical-world

[3] The colour of hope. BASF. Source: https://agriculture.basf.com/global/en/business-areas/public-health/commitment-to-public-health/methylene-blue.html

[4] Coulibaly B, Zoungrana A, Mockenhaupt FP, et al. Strong gametocytocidal effect of methylene blue-based combination therapy against falciparum malaria: a randomised controlled trial. PLoS One. 2009;4(5):e5318. https://www.ncbi.nlm.nih.gov/pubmed/19415120

[5] Schirmer RH, Coulibaly B, Stich A, et al. Methylene blue as an antimalarial agent. Redox Report. 2003;8(5):272-275. http://www.tandfonline.com/doi/abs/10.1179/135100003225002899

[6] Coulibaly B, Zoungrana A, Mockenhaupt FP, et al. Strong gametocytocidal effect of methylene blue-based combination therapy against falciparum malaria: a randomised controlled trial. PLoS One. 2009;4(5). https://www.ncbi.nlm.nih.gov/pmc/articles/PMC2673582

[7] Howland RH. Methylene blue: the long and winding road from stain to brain: part 1. J Psychosoc Nurs Ment Health Serv. 2016;54(9):21-24. https://pubmed.ncbi.nlm.nih.gov/27576224

[8] Studies on oxidation-reduction in milk: the methylene blue reduction test. Journal of Dairy Science. 1930;13(3):221-245.
https://www.sciencedirect.com/science/article/pii/S0022030230935205

[9] Mayer B, Brunner F, Schmidt K. Inhibition of nitric oxide synthesis by methylene blue. Biochem Pharmacol. 1993;45(2):367-374.
https://pubmed.ncbi.nlm.nih.gov/7679577

[10] Wrubel KM, Riha PD, Maldonado MA, McCollum D, Gonzalez-Lima F. The brain metabolic enhancer methylene blue improves discrimination learning in rats. Pharmacol Biochem Behav. 2007;86(4):712-717.
https://www.ncbi.nlm.nih.gov/pmc/articles/PMC2040387

[11] Jang DH, Nelson LS, Hoffman RS. Methylene blue in the treatment of refractory shock from an amlodipine overdose. Ann Emerg Med. 2011;58(6):565-567.
https://pubmed.ncbi.nlm.nih.gov/21546119

[12] Eroğlu L, Cağlayan B. Anxiolytic and antidepressant properties of methylene blue in animal models. Pharmacol Res. 1997;36(5):381-385.
https://pubmed.ncbi.nlm.nih.gov/9441729

[13] Barron ESG. The catalytic effect of methylene blue on the oxygen consumption of tumors and normal tissues. https://core.ac.uk/reader/7832690

[14] The effect of methylene blue on the oxygen consumption and respiratory quotient of normal and tumor tissue. John J Jares. University of Rochester School of Medicine. Source: http://www.medicinacomplementar.com.br/biblioteca/pdfs/Cancer/ca-10247.pdf

[15] Atamna H, Atamna W, Al-Eyd G, Shanower G, Dhahbi JM. Combined activation of the energy and cellular-defense pathways may explain the potent anti-senescence activity of methylene blue. Redox Biol. 2015;6:426-435.
https://www.ncbi.nlm.nih.gov/pmc/articles/PMC4588422

[16] Juffermans NP, Vervloet MG, Daemen-Gubbels CRG, Binnekade JM, de Jong M, Groeneveld ABJ. A dose-finding study of methylene blue to inhibit nitric oxide actions in the hemodynamics of human septic shock. Nitric Oxide. 2010;22(4):275-280.
https://pubmed.ncbi.nlm.nih.gov/20109575

[17] Moore T, Sharman IM, Ward RJ. The vitamin E activity of methylene blue. Biochem J. 1953;53(4):xxxi. https://pubmed.ncbi.nlm.nih.gov/13037684

[18] Gillman PK. Methylene blue is a potent monoamine oxidase inhibitor. Can J Anaesth. 2008;55(5):311-312; author reply 312.
https://pubmed.ncbi.nlm.nih.gov/18451123

[19] Wen Y, Li W, Poteet EC, et al. Alternative mitochondrial electron transfer as a novel strategy for neuroprotection. J Biol Chem. 2011;286(18):16504-16515. https://pubmed.ncbi.nlm.nih.gov/21454572

[20] Nedvídková J, Pacák K, Haluzík M, Nedvídek J, Schreiber V. The role of dopamine in methylene blue-mediated inhibition of estradiol benzoate-induced anterior pituitary hyperplasia in rats. Neurosci Lett. 2001;304(3):194-198. https://pubmed.ncbi.nlm.nih.gov/11343835

[21] Hirsch JI, Banks WL, Sullivan JS, Horsley JS. Effect of methylene blue on estrogen-receptor activity. Radiology. 1989;171(1):105-107. https://pubmed.ncbi.nlm.nih.gov/2467322

[22] Schreiber V. [Methylene blue as an endocrine modulator: interactions with thyroid hormones]. Bratisl Lek Listy. 1995;96(11):586-587. https://pubmed.ncbi.nlm.nih.gov/8624735

[23] Haluzík M, Nedvídková J, Schreiber V. Methylene blue--an endocrine modulator. Sb Lek. 1995;96(4):319-322. https://pubmed.ncbi.nlm.nih.gov/8711376

[24] Jourabi FG, Yari S, Amiri P, Heidarianpour A, Hashemi H. The ameliorative effects of methylene blue on testicular damage induced by cisplatin in rats. Andrologia. 2021;53(1):e13850. https://onlinelibrary.wiley.com/doi/abs/10.1111/and.13850

Top 10 Benefits of Methylene Blue

[1] Caroline FB, Luiza MS, Livia A, et al. Why methylene blue have to be always present in the stocking of emergency antidotes. Current Drug Targets. https://www.eurekaselect.com/node/160936/article/why-methylene-blue-have-to-be-always-present-in-the-stocking-of-emergency-antidotes

[2] Brooks MM. Methylene blue as antidote for cyanide and carbon monoxide poisoning. Journal of the American Medical Association. 1933;100(1):59-59. https://jamanetwork.com/journals/jama/article-abstract/241035

[3] Haouzi P, Gueguinou M, Sonobe T, et al. Revisiting the physiological effects of methylene blue as a treatment of cyanide intoxication. Clin Toxicol (Phila). 2018;56(9):828-840. https://pubmed.ncbi.nlm.nih.gov/29451035

[4] Joshi P, Kaya C, Surana S, et al. A novel method in decision making for the diagnosis of anterior urethral stricture: using methylene blue dye. Turk J Urol. 2017;43(4):502-506. https://www.ncbi.nlm.nih.gov/pmc/articles/PMC5687215

[5] The cinchona alkaloids and the aminoquinolines. Antimalarial Agents. Published online January 1, 2020:65-98.
https://www.sciencedirect.com/science/article/pii/B9780081012109000032

[6] The Right Chemistry: methylene blue shakes up the medical world. Montreal Gazette. 2016. Joe Schwarcz. Source:
https://montrealgazette.com/opinion/columnists/the-right-chemistry-methylene-blue-shakes-up-the-medical-world

[7] The Colour of Hope. BASF. Source:
https://agriculture.basf.com/global/en/business-areas/public-health/commitment-to-public-health/methylene-blue.html

[8] Potential health benefits of methylene blue. News Medical life sciences. Sara Ryding. Source: https://www.news-medical.net/health/Potential-Health-Benefits-of-Methylene-Blue.aspx

[9] The Colour of Hope. BASF. Source:
https://agriculture.basf.com/global/en/business-areas/public-health/commitment-to-public-health/methylene-blue.html

[10] Dicko A, Roh ME, Diawara H, et al. Efficacy and safety of primaquine and methylene blue for prevention of Plasmodium falciparum transmission in Mali: a phase 2, single-blind, randomised controlled trial. The Lancet Infectious Diseases. 2018;18(6):627-639. https://www.thelancet.com/journals/laninf/article/PIIS1473-3099(18)30044-6/fulltext

[11] Lu G, Nagbanshi M, Goldau N, et al. Efficacy and safety of methylene blue in the treatment of malaria: a systematic review. BMC Med. 2018;16(1):59.
https://pubmed.ncbi.nlm.nih.gov/29690878

[12] Gomes TF, Pedrosa MM, de Toledo ACL, et al. Bactericide effect of methylene blue associated with low-level laser therapy in Escherichia coli bacteria isolated from pressure ulcers. Lasers Med Sci. 2018;33(8):1723-1731.
https://pubmed.ncbi.nlm.nih.gov/29744751

[13] Gazel D, Tatman Otkun M, Akçalı A. In vitro activity of methylene blue and eosin methylene blue agar on colistin-resistant A. baumannii: an experimental study. J Med Microbiol. 2019;68(11):1607-1613. https://pubmed.ncbi.nlm.nih.gov/31535963

[14] Ansari MA, Fatima Z, Hameed S. Antifungal action of methylene blue involves mitochondrial dysfunction and disruption of redox and membrane homeostasis in c.

Albicans. Open Microbiol J. 2016;10:12-22.
https://pubmed.ncbi.nlm.nih.gov/27006725

[15] Wang Y, Ren K, Liao X, et al. Inactivation of Zika virus in plasma and derivatives by four different methods. J Med Virol. 2019;91(12):2059-2065.
https://pubmed.ncbi.nlm.nih.gov/31389019

[16] Papin JF, Floyd RA, Dittmer DP. Methylene blue photoinactivation abolishes West Nile virus infectivity in vivo. Antiviral Res. 2005;68(2):84-87.
https://pubmed.ncbi.nlm.nih.gov/16118025

[17] Eickmann M, Gravemann U, Handke W, et al. Inactivation of Ebola virus and Middle East respiratory syndrome coronavirus in platelet concentrates and plasma by ultraviolet C light and methylene blue plus visible light, respectively. Transfusion. 2018;58(9):2202-2207. https://www.ncbi.nlm.nih.gov/pmc/articles/PMC7169708

[18] Squillace DM, Zhao Z, Call GM, Gao J, Yao JQ. Viral inactivation of human osteochondral grafts with methylene blue and light. Cartilage. 2014;5(1):28-36.
https://www.ncbi.nlm.nih.gov/pmc/articles/PMC4297095

[19] Wong T-W, Huang H-J, Wang Y-F, Lee Y-P, Huang C-C, Yu C-K. Methylene blue-mediated photodynamic inactivation as a novel disinfectant of enterovirus 71. J Antimicrob Chemother. 2010;65(10):2176-2182.
https://pubmed.ncbi.nlm.nih.gov/20719762

[20] Methylene blue photoinactivation of RNA viruses. Antiviral Research. 2004;61(3):141-151.
https://www.sciencedirect.com/science/article/abs/pii/S0166354203002596

[21] Müller-Breitkreutz K, Mohr H. Hepatitis C and human immunodeficiency virus RNA degradation by methylene blue/light treatment of human plasma. J Med Virol. 1998;56(3):239-245. https://pubmed.ncbi.nlm.nih.gov/9783692

[22] Huang Q, Fu W-L, Chen B, Huang J-F, Zhang X, Xue Q. Inactivation of dengue virus by methylene blue/narrow bandwidth light system. J Photochem Photobiol B. 2004;77(1):39-43. https://www.ncbi.nlm.nih.gov/pmc/articles/PMC7129913

[23] Methylene blue photochemical treatment as a reliable SARS-CoV-2 plasma virus inactivation method for blood safety and convalescent plasma therapy for the COVID-19 outbreak. https://www.researchsquare.com/article/rs-17718/v1

[24] Gendrot M, Andreani J, Duflot I, et al. Methylene blue inhibits replication of SARS-CoV-2 in vitro. Int J Antimicrob Agents. 2020;56(6):106202.
https://pubmed.ncbi.nlm.nih.gov/33075512

[25] A cohort of cancer patients with no reported cases of sars-cov-s infection: the possible preventive role of methylene blue. Guerir du cancer. 2020. Source: https://guerir-du-cancer.fr/a-cohort-of-cancer-patients-with-no-reported-cases-of-sars-cov-2-infection-the-possible-preventive-role-of-methylene-blue

[26] Ajaz S, McPhail MJ, Singh KK, et al. Mitochondrial metabolic manipulation by SARS-CoV-2 in peripheral blood mononuclear cells of patients with COVID-19. American Journal of Physiology-Cell Physiology. 2020;320(1):C57-C65. https://journals.physiology.org/doi/full/10.1152/ajpcell.00426.2020

[27] Ajaz S, McPhail MJ, Singh KK, et al. Mitochondrial metabolic manipulation by SARS-CoV-2 in peripheral blood mononuclear cells of patients with COVID-19. American Journal of Physiology-Cell Physiology. 2020;320(1):C57-C65. https://journals.physiology.org/doi/full/10.1152/ajpcell.00426.2020

[28] Scigliano G, Scigliano GA. Methylene blue in COVID-19. Med Hypotheses. 2021;146:110455. https://pubmed.ncbi.nlm.nih.gov/33341032

[29] Sonntag K-C, Ryu W-I, Amirault KM, et al. Late-onset Alzheimer's disease is associated with inherent changes in bioenergetics profiles. Scientific Reports. 2017;7(1):14038. https://www.nature.com/articles/s41598-017-14420-x

[30] McCann SM, Licinio J, Wong ML, Yu WH, Karanth S, Rettorri V. The nitric oxide hypothesis of aging. Exp Gerontol. 1998;33(7-8):813-826. https://pubmed.ncbi.nlm.nih.gov/9951625

[31] McCann SM. The nitric oxide hypothesis of brain aging. Exp Gerontol. 1997;32(4-5):431-440. https://pubmed.ncbi.nlm.nih.gov/9315447

[32] Gais S, Born J. Low acetylcholine during slow-wave sleep is critical for declarative memory consolidation. PNAS. 2004;101(7):2140-2144. https://www.pnas.org/content/101/7/2140.full

[33] Shytle RD, Silver AA, Lukas RJ, Newman MB, Sheehan DV, Sanberg PR. Nicotinic acetylcholine receptors as targets for antidepressants. Mol Psychiatry. 2002;7(6):525-535. https://pubmed.ncbi.nlm.nih.gov/12140772

[34] Andreasen JT, Olsen GM, Wiborg O, Redrobe JP. Antidepressant-like effects of nicotinic acetylcholine receptor antagonists, but not agonists, in the mouse forced swim and mouse tail suspension tests. J Psychopharmacol. 2009;23(7):797-804. https://pubmed.ncbi.nlm.nih.gov/18583432

[35] Sawada Y, Nakamura M, Bito T, et al. Cholinergic urticaria: studies on the muscarinic cholinergic receptor M3 in anhidrotic and hypohidrotic skin. J Invest Dermatol. 2010;130(11):2683-2686. https://pubmed.ncbi.nlm.nih.gov/20613776

[36] Sawada Y, Nakamura M, Bito T, et al. Decreased expression of acetylcholine esterase in cholinergic urticaria with hypohidrosis or anhidrosis. J Invest Dermatol. 2014;134(1):276-279. https://pubmed.ncbi.nlm.nih.gov/23748235

[37] Abdulla SAM, Dietrich EL, Syed MN, et al. Methylene blue inhibits the function of α7-nicotinic acetylcholine receptors. CNS & Neurological Disorders - Drug Targets. https://www.eurekaselect.com/104080/article

[38] Schelter BO, Shiells H, Baddeley TC, et al. Concentration-dependent activity of hydromethylthionine on cognitive decline and brain atrophy in mild to moderate alzheimer's disease. J Alzheimers Dis. 2019;72(3):931-946. https://pubmed.ncbi.nlm.nih.gov/31658058

[39] New study by TauRx shows a minimum dose of hydromethylthionine could slow cognitive decline and brain atrophy in mild-to-moderate Alzheimer's disease. PRNewswire. 2019. Source: https://www.prnewswire.com/news-releases/new-study-by-taurx-shows-a-minimum-dose-of-hydromethylthionine-could-slow-cognitive-decline-and-brain-atrophy-in-mild-to-moderate-alzheimers-disease-300965395.html

[40] Soeda Y, Saito M, Maeda S, et al. Methylene blue inhibits formation of tau fibrils but not of granular tau oligomers: a plausible key to understanding failure of a clinical trial for alzheimer's disease. J Alzheimers Dis. 2019;68(4):1677-1686. https://pubmed.ncbi.nlm.nih.gov/30909223

[41] Necula M, Breydo L, Milton S, et al. Methylene blue inhibits amyloid aβ oligomerization by promoting fibrillization. Biochemistry. 2007;46(30):8850-8860. https://pubs.acs.org/doi/10.1021/bi700411k

[42] TauRx Alzheimer's drug ltmx fails in large study although some benefit seen. NBC News. Source: https://www.nbcnews.com/health/health-news/taurx-alzheimer-s-drug-lmtx-fails-large-study-although-some-n617746

[43] Second phase II study results for anti-tau Alzheimer's treatment released. Alzheimer's research UK. 2017. Source: https://www.alzheimersresearchuk.org/second-phase-iii-study-results-anti-tau-alzheimers-treatment-released

[44] Wrubel KM, Riha PD, Maldonado MA, McCollum D, Gonzalez-Lima F. The brain metabolic enhancer methylene blue improves discrimination learning in rats. Pharmacol Biochem Behav. 2007;86(4):712-717. https://www.ncbi.nlm.nih.gov/pmc/articles/PMC2040387

[45] Atamna H, Nguyen A, Schultz C, et al. Methylene blue delays cellular senescence and enhances key mitochondrial biochemical pathways. FASEB J. 2008;22(3):703-712. https://www.ncbi.nlm.nih.gov/pubmed/17928358

[46] Potential alzheimer's, parkinson's cure found in century-old drug. ScienceDaily. Source: https://www.sciencedaily.com/releases/2008/08/080818101335.htm

[47] Glucose deprivation in the brain sets stage for Alzheimer's disease, Temple study shows. EurekAlert! Source: https://www.eurekalert.org/pub_releases/2017-01/tuhs-gdi012717.php

[48] Choudhury GR, Winters A, Rich RM, et al. Methylene blue protects astrocytes against glucose oxygen deprivation by improving cellular respiration. PLOS ONE. 2015;10(4):e0123096. https://journals.plos.org/plosone/article?id=10.1371/journal.pone.0123096

[49] Yang L, Youngblood H, Wu C, Zhang Q. Mitochondria as a target for neuroprotection: role of methylene blue and photobiomodulation. Translational Neurodegeneration. 2020;9(1):19. https://translationalneurodegeneration.biomedcentral.com/articles/10.1186/s40035-020-00197-z

[50] Rodriguez P, Zhou W, Barrett DW, et al. Multimodal randomized functional mr imaging of the effects of methylene blue in the human brain. Radiology. 2016;281(2):516-526. https://pubs.rsna.org/doi/10.1148/radiol.2016152893

[51] Methylene blue shows promise for improving short-term memory: Study in humans. ScienceDaily. https://www.sciencedaily.com/releases/2016/06/160628072028.htm

[52] Lin A-L, Poteet E, Du F, et al. Methylene blue as a cerebral metabolic and hemodynamic enhancer. PLOS ONE. 2012;7(10):e46585. https://journals.plos.org/plosone/article?id=10.1371/journal.pone.0046585

[53] James BM, Li Q, Luo L, Kendrick KM. Aged neuronal nitric oxide knockout mice show preserved olfactory learning in both social recognition and odor-conditioning tasks. Front Cell Neurosci. 2015;9:105. https://pubmed.ncbi.nlm.nih.gov/25870540

[54] Cowen PJ, Browning M. What has serotonin to do with depression? World Psychiatry. 2015;14(2):158-160. https://www.ncbi.nlm.nih.gov/pmc/articles/PMC4471964

[55] Teng T, Shively CA, Li X, et al. Chronic unpredictable mild stress produces depressive-like behavior, hypercortisolemia, and metabolic dysfunction in adolescent

cynomolgus monkeys. Translational Psychiatry. 2021;11(1):1-9.
https://www.nature.com/articles/s41398-020-01132-6

56 Hinnouho G-M, Singh-Manoux A, Gueguen A, et al. Metabolically healthy obesity and depressive symptoms: 16-year follow-up of the Gazel cohort study. PLOS ONE. 2017;12(4):e0174678.
https://journals.plos.org/plosone/article?id=10.1371/journal.pone.0174678

57 Gowey MA, Khodneva Y, Tison SE, et al. Depressive symptoms, perceived stress, and metabolic health: The REGARDS study. International Journal of Obesity. 2019;43(3):615-632. https://www.nature.com/articles/s41366-018-0270-3

58 Major depression leaves metabolic signature. Medical News Today. 2015. James McIntosh. Source: https://www.medicalnewstoday.com/articles/292842

59 Women and depression. Harvard health publishing. 2011. Source: https://www.health.harvard.edu/womens-health/women-and-depression

60 Salk RH, Hyde JS, Abramson LY. Gender differences in depression in representative national samples: Meta-analyses of diagnoses and symptoms. Psychol Bull. 2017;143(8):783-822. https://pubmed.ncbi.nlm.nih.gov/28447828/

61 Hiroi R, McDevitt RA, Neumaier JF. Estrogen selectively increases tryptophan hydroxylase-2 mRNA expression in distinct subregions of rat midbrain raphe nucleus: association between gene expression and anxiety behavior in the open field. Biol Psychiatry. 2006;60(3):288-295. https://pubmed.ncbi.nlm.nih.gov/16458260

62 Qureshi AC, Bahri A, Breen LA, et al. The influence of the route of oestrogen administration on serum levels of cortisol-binding globulin and total cortisol. Clin Endocrinol (Oxf). 2007;66(5):632-635. https://pubmed.ncbi.nlm.nih.gov/17492949

63 Nevzati E, Shafighi M, Bakhtian KD, Treiber H, Fandino J, Fathi AR. Estrogen induces nitric oxide production via nitric oxide synthase activation in endothelial cells. Acta Neurochir Suppl. 2015;120:141-145. https://pubmed.ncbi.nlm.nih.gov/25366614

64 Kudlow P, Cha DS, Carvalho AF, McIntyre RS. Nitric oxide and major depressive disorder: pathophysiology and treatment implications. Curr Mol Med. 2016;16(2):206-215. https://pubmed.ncbi.nlm.nih.gov/26812915

65 Gao S-F, Lu Y-R, Shi L-G, et al. Nitric oxide synthase and nitric oxide alterations in chronically stressed rats: a model for nitric oxide in major depressive disorder. Psychoneuroendocrinology. 2014;47:136-140.
https://pubmed.ncbi.nlm.nih.gov/25001963

[66] Akpinar A, Yaman GB, Demirdas A, Onal S. Possible role of adrenomedullin and nitric oxide in major depression. Prog Neuropsychopharmacol Biol Psychiatry. 2013;46:120-125. https://pubmed.ncbi.nlm.nih.gov/23867466

[67] Joca SRL, Guimarães FS. Inhibition of neuronal nitric oxide synthase in the rat hippocampus induces antidepressant-like effects. Psychopharmacology (Berl). 2006;185(3):298-305. https://pubmed.ncbi.nlm.nih.gov/16518647

[68] Naylor GJ, Smith AH, Connelly P. A controlled trial of methylene blue in severe depressive illness. Biol Psychiatry. 1987;22(5):657-659. https://pubmed.ncbi.nlm.nih.gov/3555627

[69] Naylor GJ, Martin B, Hopwood SE, Watson Y. A two-year double-blind crossover trial of the prophylactic effect of methylene blue in manic-depressive psychosis. Biol Psychiatry. 1986;21(10):915-920. https://pubmed.ncbi.nlm.nih.gov/3091097

[70] Alda M, McKinnon M, Blagdon R, et al. Methylene blue treatment for residual symptoms of bipolar disorder: randomised crossover study. Br J Psychiatry. 2017;210(1):54-60. https://pubmed.ncbi.nlm.nih.gov/27284082

[71] Telch MJ, Bruchey AK, Rosenfield D, et al. Effects of post-session administration of methylene blue on fear extinction and contextual memory in adults with claustrophobia. Am J Psychiatry. 2014;171(10):1091-1098. https://pubmed.ncbi.nlm.nih.gov/25018057

[72] Auchter AM, Shumake J, Gonzalez-Lima F, Monfils MH. Preventing the return of fear using reconsolidation updating and methylene blue is differentially dependent on extinction learning. Sci Rep. 2017;7:46071. https://pubmed.ncbi.nlm.nih.gov/28397861

[73] Zoellner LA, Telch M, Foa EB, et al. Enhancing extinction learning in posttraumatic stress disorder with brief daily imaginal exposure and methylene blue: a randomized controlled trial. J Clin Psychiatry. 2017;78(7):e782-e789. https://pubmed.ncbi.nlm.nih.gov/28686823

[74] Alda M. Methylene blue in the treatment of neuropsychiatric disorders. CNS Drugs. 2019;33(8):719-725. https://pubmed.ncbi.nlm.nih.gov/31144270

[75] What are the treatments for autism WebMD. 2020. Renee A. Alli, MD. Source: https://www.webmd.com/brain/autism/understanding-autism-treatment

[76] Giulivi C, Zhang Y-F, Omanska-Klusek A, et al. Mitochondrial dysfunction in autism. JAMA. 2010;304(21):2389. https://jamanetwork.com/journals/jama/fullarticle/186999

[77] Children with autism have mitochondrial dysfunction, study finds. Science Daily. 2010. Source: https://www.sciencedaily.com/releases/2010/11/101130161521.htm

[78] Chakraborty P, Carpenter KLH, Major S, et al. Gastrointestinal problems are associated with increased repetitive behaviors but not social communication difficulties in young children with autism spectrum disorders. Autism. 2021;25(2):405-415. https://journals.sagepub.com/doi/10.1177/1362361320959503

[79] Autism study suggests connection between repetitive behaviors, gut problems. Science Daily. 2020. Source: https://www.sciencedaily.com/releases/2020/12/201203094542.htm

[80] Lipopolysaccharide-induced inflammation and perinatal brain injury. Seminars in Fetal and Neonatal Medicine. 2006;11(5):343-353. https://www.sciencedirect.com/science/article/pii/S1744165X06000448

[81] Zhao J, Bi W, Xiao S, et al. Neuroinflammation induced by lipopolysaccharide causes cognitive impairment in mice. Scientific Reports. 2019;9(1):5790. https://www.nature.com/articles/s41598-019-42286-8

[82] Singal A, Tirkey N, Pilkhwal S, Chopra K. Green tea (Camellia sinensis) extract ameliorates endotoxin induced sickness behavior and liver damage in rats. Phytother Res. 2006;20(2):125-129. https://pubmed.ncbi.nlm.nih.gov/16444665

[83] Yirmiya R, Pollak Y, Morag M, et al. Illness, cytokines, and depression. Ann N Y Acad Sci. 2000;917:478-487. https://pubmed.ncbi.nlm.nih.gov/11268375

[84] Marvel FA, Chen C-C, Badr N, Gaykema RPA, Goehler LE. Reversible inactivation of the dorsal vagal complex blocks lipopolysaccharide-induced social withdrawal and c-Fos expression in central autonomic nuclei. Brain Behav Immun. 2004;18(2):123-134. https://pubmed.ncbi.nlm.nih.gov/14759590

[85] Potentiation of mercury-induced nephrotoxicity by endotoxin in the Sprague–Dawley rat. Toxicology. 2000;149(2-3):75-87. https://www.sciencedirect.com/science/article/pii/S0300483X0000233X

[86] Altered glutathione homeostasis in animals prenatally exposed to lipopolysaccharide. Neurochemistry International. 2007;50(4):671-680. https://www.sciencedirect.com/science/article/pii/S0197018607000186

[87] Hou Y, Xie G, Liu X, et al. Minocycline protects against lipopolysaccharide-induced cognitive impairment in mice. Psychopharmacology (Berl). 2016;233(5):905-916. https://pubmed.ncbi.nlm.nih.gov/26645224

[88] Yin S, Shao J, Wang X, et al. Methylene blue exerts rapid neuroprotective effects on lipopolysaccharide-induced behavioral deficits in mice. Behav Brain Res. 2019;356:288-294. https://pubmed.ncbi.nlm.nih.gov/30195022

[89] Huang TH, Lu YC, Kao CT. Low-level diode laser therapy reduces lipopolysaccharide (Lps)-induced bone cell inflammation. Lasers Med Sci. 2012;27(3):621-627. https://pubmed.ncbi.nlm.nih.gov/22002329

[90] Effects of activated charcoal and zeolite on serum lipopolysaccharides and some inflammatory biomarkers levels in experimentally induced subacute ruminal acidosis in lambs. Turkish journal of veterinary and animal sciences. 2020. Source: https://journals.tubitak.gov.tr/veterinary/issues/vet-20-44-4/vet-44-4-10-2001-93.pdf

[91] Frolkis VV, Nikolaev VG, Paramonova GI, et al. Effect of enterosorption on animal lifespan. Biomater Artif Cells Artif Organs. 1989;17(3):341-351. https://pubmed.ncbi.nlm.nih.gov/2479433

[92] Frye RE, Rossignol DA. Mitochondrial dysfunction can connect the diverse medical symptoms associated with autism spectrum disorders. Pediatr Res. 2011;69(5 Pt 2):41R-47R. https://www.ncbi.nlm.nih.gov/pmc/articles/PMC3179978

[93] Guevara-Campos J, González-Guevara L, Puig-Alcaraz C, Cauli O. Autism spectrum disorders associated to a deficiency of the enzymes of the mitochondrial respiratory chain. Metab Brain Dis. 2013;28(4):605-612. https://pubmed.ncbi.nlm.nih.gov/23839164

[94] Goh S, Dong Z, Zhang Y, DiMauro S, Peterson BS. Mitochondrial dysfunction as a neurobiological subtype of autism spectrum disorder: evidence from brain imaging. JAMA Psychiatry. 2014;71(6):665-671. https://pubmed.ncbi.nlm.nih.gov/24718932

[95] Frye RE, Rose S, Slattery J, MacFabe DF. Gastrointestinal dysfunction in autism spectrum disorder: the role of the mitochondria and the enteric microbiome. Microb Ecol Health Dis. 2015;26:27458. https://pubmed.ncbi.nlm.nih.gov/25956238

[96] Siddiqui MF, Elwell C, Johnson MH. Mitochondrial dysfunction in autism spectrum disorders. Autism Open Access. 2016;6(5). https://www.ncbi.nlm.nih.gov/pmc/articles/PMC5137782

[97] Mitochondrial dysfunction in autism spectrum disorder: unique abnormalities and targeted treatments. Seminars in Pediatric Neurology. 2020;35:100829. https://www.sciencedirect.com/science/article/pii/S1071909120300401

[98] Lin A-L, Poteet E, Du F, et al. Methylene blue as a cerebral metabolic and hemodynamic enhancer. PLOS ONE. 2012;7(10):e46585. https://journals.plos.org/plosone/article?id=10.1371/journal.pone.0046585

[99] Atamna H, Nguyen A, Schultz C, et al. Methylene blue delays cellular senescence and enhances key mitochondrial biochemical pathways. FASEB J. 2008;22(3):703-712. https://www.ncbi.nlm.nih.gov/pubmed/17928358

[100] Ueber schmerzstillende wirkung des methylenblaus (Pp. 493-494). Von ehrlich, paul & leppmann, a. (1890): | antiq. F. -d. Söhn - medicusbooks. Com. https://www.zvab.com/Ueber-schmerzstillende-Wirkung-Methylenblaus-pp.493-494-Ehrlich/1239519850/bd

[101] Sim H-L, Tan K-Y. Randomized single-blind clinical trial of intradermal methylene blue on pain reduction after open diathermy haemorrhoidectomy. Colorectal Dis. 2014;16(8):O283-287. https://pubmed.ncbi.nlm.nih.gov/24506265

[102] Miclescu AA, Svahn M, Gordh TE. Evaluation of the protein biomarkers and the analgesic response to systemic methylene blue in patients with refractory neuropathic pain: a double-blind, controlled study. J Pain Res. 2015;8:387-397. https://www.ncbi.nlm.nih.gov/pmc/articles/PMC4509536

[103] Roldan CJ, Chung M, Feng L, Bruera E. Methylene blue for the treatment of intractable pain from oral mucositis related to cancer treatment: an uncontrolled cohort. J Natl Compr Canc Netw. Published online January 4, 2021:1-7. https://pubmed.ncbi.nlm.nih.gov/33395626

[104] Li X, Tang C, Wang J, et al. Methylene blue relieves the development of osteoarthritis by upregulating lncRNA MEG3. Exp Ther Med. 2018;15(4):3856-3864. https://www.ncbi.nlm.nih.gov/pmc/articles/PMC5863598

[105] Cohen N, Robinson D, Ben-Ezzer J, et al. Reduced NO accumulation in arthrotic cartilage by exposure to methylene blue. Acta Orthop Scand. 2000;71(6):630-636. https://pubmed.ncbi.nlm.nih.gov/11145393

[106] Pradhan AA, Bertels Z, Akerman S. Targeted nitric oxide synthase inhibitors for migraine. Neurotherapeutics. 2018;15(2):391-401. https://www.ncbi.nlm.nih.gov/pmc/articles/PMC5935643

[107] Peng B, Pang X, Wu Y, Zhao C, Song X. A randomized placebo-controlled trial of intradiscal methylene blue injection for the treatment of chronic discogenic low back pain. Pain. 2010;149(1):124-129. https://pubmed.ncbi.nlm.nih.gov/20167430

[108] Surprisingly effective back pain injection: intradiscal methylene blue. Pain Science. 2010. Source: https://www.painscience.com/biblio/surprisingly-effective-back-pain-injection--intradiscal-methylene-blue.html

[109] Glenn CL, Wang WY, Morris BJ. Different frequencies of inducible nitric oxide synthase genotypes in older hypertensives. Hypertension. 1999;33(4):927-932. https://pubmed.ncbi.nlm.nih.gov/10205225

[110] Mungrue IN, Gros R, You X, et al. Cardiomyocyte overexpression of iNOS in mice results in peroxynitrite generation, heart block, and sudden death. J Clin Invest. 2002;109(6):735-743. https://www.ncbi.nlm.nih.gov/pmc/articles/PMC150906

[111] Kim JH, Bugaj LJ, Oh YJ, et al. Arginase inhibition restores NOS coupling and reverses endothelial dysfunction and vascular stiffness in old rats. J Appl Physiol (1985). 2009;107(4):1249-1257. https://pubmed.ncbi.nlm.nih.gov/19661445

[112] Smith CJ, Santhanam L, Bruning RS, Stanhewicz A, Berkowitz DE, Holowatz LA. Upregulation of inducible nitric oxide synthase contributes to attenuated cutaneous vasodilation in essential hypertensive humans. Hypertension. 2011;58(5):935-942. https://pubmed.ncbi.nlm.nih.gov/21931069

[113] Van der Loo B, Labugger R, Skepper JN, et al. Enhanced peroxynitrite formation is associated with vascular aging. J Exp Med. 2000;192(12):1731-1744. https://pubmed.ncbi.nlm.nih.gov/11120770

[114] Peluffo G, Radi R. Biochemistry of protein tyrosine nitration in cardiovascular pathology. Cardiovasc Res. 2007;75(2):291-302. https://pubmed.ncbi.nlm.nih.gov/17544386

[115] Santhanam L, Lim HK, Lim HK, et al. Inducible NO synthase dependent S-nitrosylation and activation of arginase1 contribute to age-related endothelial dysfunction. Circ Res. 2007;101(7):692-702. https://pubmed.ncbi.nlm.nih.gov/17704205

[116] Lomniczi A, Cebral E, Canteros G, McCann SM, Rettori V. Methylene blue inhibits the increase of inducible nitric oxide synthase activity induced by stress and lipopolysaccharide in the medial basal hypothalamus of rats. Neuroimmunomodulation. 2000;8(3):122-127. https://pubmed.ncbi.nlm.nih.gov/11124577

[117] McCann SM, Mastronardi C, de Laurentiis A, Rettori V. The nitric oxide theory of aging revisited. Ann N Y Acad Sci. 2005;1057:64-84. https://pubmed.ncbi.nlm.nih.gov/16399888

[118] Plumb B, Parker A, Wong P. Feeling blue with metformin-associated lactic acidosis. BMJ Case Rep. 2013;2013. https://pubmed.ncbi.nlm.nih.gov/23456165

[119] Duicu OM, Privistirescu A, Wolf A, et al. Methylene blue improves mitochondrial respiration and decreases oxidative stress in a substrate-dependent manner in diabetic

rat hearts. Can J Physiol Pharmacol. 2017;95(11):1376-1382.
https://pubmed.ncbi.nlm.nih.gov/28738167

[120] Highet DM, West ES. The effect of methylene blue in preventing alloxan diabetes
and in lowering the blood sugar of alloxan-diabetic rats. J Biol Chem. 1949;178(1):521.
https://pubmed.ncbi.nlm.nih.gov/18112136

[121] Hao J, Zhang H, Yu J, Chen X, Yang L. Methylene blue attenuates diabetic
retinopathy by inhibiting nlrp3 inflammasome activation in stz-induced diabetic rats.
Ocul Immunol Inflamm. 2019;27(5):836-843.
https://pubmed.ncbi.nlm.nih.gov/29608341

[122] Highet DM, West ES. The effect of methylene blue in preventing alloxan diabetes
and in lowering the blood sugar of alloxan-diabetic rats. J Biol Chem. 1949;178(1):521.
https://pubmed.ncbi.nlm.nih.gov/18112136

[123] Vander Heiden MG, Cantley LC, Thompson CB. Understanding the warburg effect:
the metabolic requirements of cell proliferation. Science. 2009;324(5930):1029-1033.
https://www.ncbi.nlm.nih.gov/pmc/articles/PMC2849637

[124] Israel BA, Schaeffer WI. Cytoplasmic suppression of malignancy. In Vitro Cell Dev
Biol. 1987;23(9):627-632. https://pubmed.ncbi.nlm.nih.gov/3654482

[125] Milo GE, Shuler CF, Lee H, Casto BC. A conundrum in molecular toxicology:
molecular and biological changes during neoplastic transformation of human cells. Cell
Biol Toxicol. 1995;11(6):329-345. https://pubmed.ncbi.nlm.nih.gov/8788209

[126] Gallo O, Masini E, Morbidelli L, et al. Role of nitric oxide in angiogenesis and
tumor progression in head and neck cancer. J Natl Cancer Inst. 1998;90(8):587-596.
https://pubmed.ncbi.nlm.nih.gov/9554441

[127] Dillekås H, Rogers MS, Straume O. Are 90% of deaths from cancer caused by
metastases? Cancer Medicine. 2019;8(12):5574-5576.
https://onlinelibrary.wiley.com/doi/full/10.1002/cam4.2474

[128] Vidal MJ, Zocchi MR, Poggi A, Pellagatta F, Chierchia SL. Involvement of nitric
oxide in tumor cell adhesion to cytokine-activated endothelial cells. Eur PMC. 1992.
Source: http://europepmc.org/article/MED/1282956

[129] Barron ESG. The catalytic effect of methylene blue on the oxygen consumption of
tumors and normal tissues. https://core.ac.uk/reader/7832690

[130] Dos Santos AF, Terra LF, Wailemann RAM, et al. Methylene blue photodynamic
therapy induces selective and massive cell death in human breast cancer cells. BMC

Cancer. 2017;17(1):194.
https://bmccancer.biomedcentral.com/articles/10.1186/s12885-017-3179-7

[131] Dong DW, Srinivasan S, Guha M, Avadhani NG. Defects in cytochrome c oxidase expression induce a metabolic shift to glycolysis and carcinogenesis. Genom Data. 2015;6:99-107. https://pubmed.ncbi.nlm.nih.gov/26697345

[132] Salehpour F, Mahmoudi J, Kamari F, Sadigh-Eteghad S, Rasta SH, Hamblin MR. Brain photobiomodulation therapy: a narrative review. Mol Neurobiol. 2018;55(8):6601-6636. https://pubmed.ncbi.nlm.nih.gov/29327206

[133] Tardivo JP, Del Giglio A, de Oliveira CS, et al. Methylene blue in photodynamic therapy: From basic mechanisms to clinical applications. Photodiagnosis Photodyn Ther. 2005;2(3):175-191. https://pubmed.ncbi.nlm.nih.gov/25048768

The Methylene Blue Battery

[1] Kosswattaarachchi AM, Cook TR. Repurposing the industrial dye methylene blue as an active component for redox flow batteries. ChemElectroChem. 2018;5(22):3437-3442. https://chemistry-europe.onlinelibrary.wiley.com/doi/abs/10.1002/celc.201801097

[2] This bright blue dye is found in fabric. Could it also power batteries? University at Buffalo. 2018. Charlotte Hsu. Source: http://www.buffalo.edu/news/releases/2018/08/026.html

Methylene Blue for Dogs, Cats, Cows, Fish and Horses

[1] Methylene blue – Veterinary Systemic. The US Pharmacopeial Convention. 2008. Source: https://cdn.ymaws.com/www.aavpt.org/resource/resmgr/imported/methyleneBlue.pdf

[2] Pereira LM, Vigato-Ferreira IC, DE Luca G, Bronzon DA Costa CM, Yatsuda AP. Evaluation of methylene blue, pyrimethamine and its combination on an in vitro Neospora caninum model. Parasitology. 2017;144(6):827-833. https://pubmed.ncbi.nlm.nih.gov/28073383

[3] Van Dijk S, Lobsteyn AJ, Wensing T, Breukink HJ. Treatment of nitrate intoxication in a cow. Vet Rec. 1983;112(12):272-274. https://pubmed.ncbi.nlm.nih.gov/6845603

[4] Sellera FP, Gargano RG, Dos Anjos C, da Silva Baptista M, Ribeiro MS, Pogliani FC. Methylene blue-mediated antimicrobial photodynamic therapy: A novel strategy for

digital dermatitis-associated sole ulcer in a cow - A case report. Photodiagnosis Photodyn Ther. 2018;24:121-122. https://pubmed.ncbi.nlm.nih.gov/30217667

[5] Jaffey JA, Harmon MR, Villani NA, et al. Long-term treatment with methylene blue in a dog with hereditary methemoglobinemia caused by cytochrome b5 reductase deficiency. Journal of Veterinary Internal Medicine. 2017;31(6):1860-1865. https://onlinelibrary.wiley.com/doi/10.1111/jvim.14843

[6] Rumbeiha WK, Oehme FW. Methylene blue can be used to treat methemoglobinemia in cats without inducing Heinz body hemolytic anemia. Vet Hum Toxicol. 1992;34(2):120-122. https://pubmed.ncbi.nlm.nih.gov/1509670

Safety, Dose, and Where to Get Methylene Blue?

[1] Ginimuge PR, Jyothi SD. Methylene blue: revisited. J Anaesthesiol Clin Pharmacol. 2010;26(4):517-520. https://www.ncbi.nlm.nih.gov/pmc/articles/PMC3087269

[2] Rojas JC, Bruchey AK, Gonzalez-Lima F. Neurometabolic mechanisms for memory enhancement and neuroprotection of methylene blue. Prog Neurobiol. 2012;96(1):32-45. https://www.ncbi.nlm.nih.gov/pmc/articles/PMC3265679

[3] Kamat JP, Devasagayam TP. Methylene blue plus light-induced lipid peroxidation in rat liver microsomes: inhibition by nicotinamide (Vitamin b3) and other antioxidants. Chem Biol Interact. 1996;99(1-3):1-16. https://pubmed.ncbi.nlm.nih.gov/8620561

[4] Rojas JC, Bruchey AK, Gonzalez-Lima F. Neurometabolic mechanisms for memory enhancement and neuroprotection of methylene blue. Prog Neurobiol. 2012;96(1):32-45. https://www.ncbi.nlm.nih.gov/pmc/articles/PMC3265679

[5] Ng BKW, Cameron AJD. The role of methylene blue in serotonin syndrome: a systematic review. Psychosomatics. 2010;51(3):194-200. https://pubmed.ncbi.nlm.nih.gov/20484716

[6] Oz M, Lorke DE, Petroianu GA. Methylene blue and Alzheimer's disease. Biochem Pharmacol. 2009;78(8):927-932. https://pubmed.ncbi.nlm.nih.gov/19433072

[7] Methylene Blue. Maryland Poison Center. February 2015. Source: https://www.mdpoison.com/media/SOP/mdpoisoncom/ToxTidbits/2015/February%202015%20ToxTidbits.pdf

[8] Ginimuge PR, Jyothi SD. Methylene blue: revisited. J Anaesthesiol Clin Pharmacol. 2010;26(4):517-520. https://www.ncbi.nlm.nih.gov/pmc/articles/PMC3087269

Printed by Libri Plureos GmbH in Hamburg,
Germany